DEEP

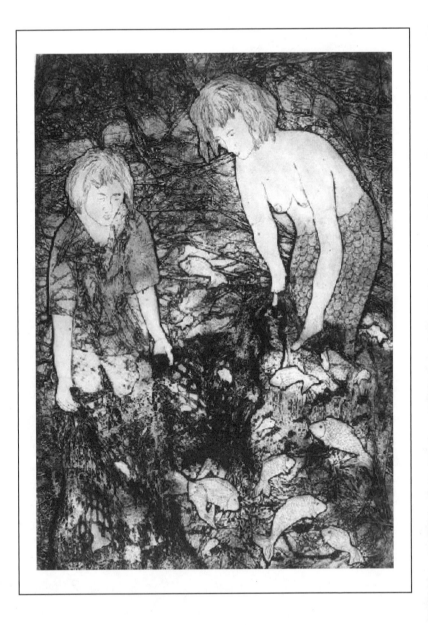

DEEP

Real Life with
Spinal Cord Injury

Marcy Epstein and Travar Pettway,

Editors

The University of Michigan Press

Ann Arbor

Published by the University of Michigan Press 2007
Copyright © 2006 by the University of Michigan
All rights reserved
Published in the United States of America by
The University of Michigan Press
Manufactured in the United States of America
⊚ Printed on acid-free paper

2010   2009   2008   2007   4   3   2   1

U.S. CIP data applied for.

ISBN-13: 978-0-472-03251-8
ISBN-10: 0-472-03251-8

For Julie

Roar . . .

FOREWORD

On behalf of my colleagues of the University of Michigan Model Systems for Spinal Cord Injury Care, I am pleased to make the opening remark for this volume, *Deep: Real Life with Spinal Cord Injury*. Reflecting research and partnership among scientists, health providers, and people in our community, this project fits into the larger picture of excellence that we wish to accomplish in all dimensions of our health system: groundbreaking and dedicated research, compassionate clinical care, progressive education, and a welcoming environment that includes community with people with disabilities. In *Deep*, the writers and editors of this book realize this mission with accuracy and clarity.

Denise G. Tate, PhD, ABPP
Director of Research
June 28, 2006

CONTENTS

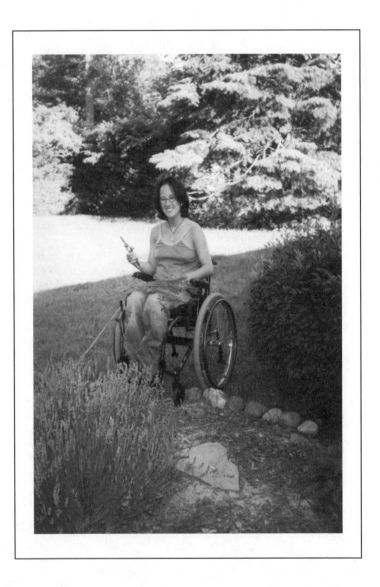

INTRODUCTION

The American psychologist and writer William James once wrote: "Our life is always deeper than we know, is always more divine than it seems, and hence we are able to survive degradations and despairs which otherwise must engulf us." The essays you are about to read embrace this depth of life. On a daily basis as people with spinal cord injuries, we swim through tremendous depth, and sometimes depths, inspired by things, people, and forces around us. Engulfed as we can become, we can also speak out from these depths, mapping the ways for other people with like injuries and others who curiously explore life. The essays to follow consist of layer upon layer of reflection, reflections by men and women who, like some of you, survive injury and live to tell about it.

We are counting on a variety of responses to these essays, since they vary in tone, style, theme, and approach. To create depth suggests the excavation of layers which draft after draft of writing often feels like. Our authors search for James' meaning and also research common themes and misconceptions, chiseling away at existing structures of expression and mining among strata of meaning. The fullness of meaning is still only realized in you, the reader. In this sense, you are the final arbiter of each work's depth. It is our hope that readers of *Deep* will find unexpected richness in the worlds we occupy but do not intensely or routinely probe.

This is also how our experiences, narrated consciously over the course of many months, can aide the understanding of others: other people with our disabilities, non-disabled others in our families, support networks, health circles, and research enterprises. Narratives have long been used to support scientific (knowledge seeking) endeavors by describing patient experiences or histories; orally told, such narratives communicate our reaction to the world as people with spinal cord injuries. We hope all these reading audiences will also dig deeply to fulfill the meaning of each piece.

We intend for these essays to represent whole lives, the thoughts and ontology (the study of unfolding being-ness) of people with spinal cord injuries. This book represents *science* in the qualitative sense of the term. Its contents illumine human experiences that intersect closely with scientific practices— biological, technical, medical, psychological. The movement in rehabilitation toward "spiritual-biopsychosocial" models of disabilities in the social, health, and medical sciences surely supports the relevance of each essay. Furthermore, this text comes about as a result of rigorous methodological research in disability and rehabilitation at the University of Michigan, specifically in a relatively new substratum of qualitative methodology called *narrative research*.

Narrative research began in the humanities and social sciences in the second half of the twentieth century and is growing now in the trans-disciplinary area of disability studies. We are trying to translate as many stories as possible by people with disabilities so that scientists can hear us. Until this year, with Simi Linton's *My Body Politic* (University of Michigan Press, 2005), the field had not yet seen an excellent, full-length exploration of narrative and spinal cord injury. A clinical psychologist by training, Linton thoughtfully and wittily traces her life before and following SCI within the social and political weave of America. Our narratives also inform theories of disability in the humanities, critiquing medicine for its historical objectification of disabled people; notably in this category of narrative research are G. Thomas Couser's "counter-narratives of biomedicine" in *Recovering Bodies: Illness, Disability, and Life Narrative* (University of Wisconsin Press, 1997) and David Mitchell and Sharon Snyder's collection of narrative interpretations about disability, *Narrative Prosthesis: Disability and the Dependencies of Discourse* (University of Michigan Press, 2001).

This collection joins two other useful texts of stories by survivors of spinal cord injuries. Jonathan Cole's *Still Lives: Narratives of Spinal Cord Injury* (Bradford Books, 2004) follows the stories of twelve people with quadriplegia. They reflect on the absence of movement and sensation in their bodies. Gary Karp and Stanley D. Klein's *From There to Here: Stories of Adjustment to Spinal Cord Injury* (No Limits Communication, 2004) is another popular text dedicated to a wide assortment of SCI topics, including some excellent attention to physical activity after SCI.

Our volume is more slender and defined than either of these worthy reads, less physical, lighter to carry yet weighty in establishing a relationship between readers and writers with SCI. Rather than focus on the medical experiences or body differences, this book plunges into the depth and depths of the human lives into which SCI enters, our philosophical and ontological issues. We look here for things that matter to us. *Deep* has been designed to be read not only for information but also specifically for the contemplation of our contributors. This book represents an experiment among usual people who become disabled, then author in a conscious, constructive manner.

Participatory Action Research (PAR) approximates the methodology we developed in this project, for PAR devotes itself to the improvement and specification of knowledge, based on the inclusion and activation of people with disabilities at every stage of the scientific process. PAR has also grown within rehabilitation science recently, injecting SCI-related professional communities with a healthy analytical and ethical infusion of disability self-representation.

Rarely and more rarely do rehabilitation research organizations treat people with disabilities merely as objects of study or bodies that are so-called broken or abnormal. In Model SCI Care Systems and other progressive research groups, we are learning within the scientific community the tremendous importance of returning the authority of our experiences to us.

This authority of knowledge about life with spinal cord injury is something our community needs. PAR is not a panacea for rehabilitation nor for people with spinal cord injuries who are still developing their own sense of authority. There's the practical problem in the recruitment, retention, accreditation, and acceptance of scientists with disabilities, particularly of scientists of color who have disabilities. As recently as June 2006 at a roundtable on a "new disability science" at the Society for Disability Studies in Washington, DC, we are still hammering out problems with PAR, such as the ownership and authorship of scientific study of SCI.

In the case of *Deep*, we have adapted a different and dialogic method of narrative research called Participatory *Authorized* Research. This PAR redistributes authority within the reporting relationship between those who collect and analyze information and those whose lives are "translated" for qualitative research, to borrow from Stephen Tingus, Director of the National Institute for Disability Research and Rehabilitation. For this sort of PAR, we emphasize being "participating authors" and "authorizing" or "authoritative participants." We look to "participating authors" with disabilities to write, analyze, and authorize our research into deep matters for people with SCI. All participating authors—regardless of demographics or backgrounds—are situated within their essays as the scientific leads on their topics. A last significant distinction of this PAR method is that participation in *Deep* led to publication in this volume, rather than a more traditional experimental article. We chose to write a monograph of collective voices instead of writing a journal article concerning "what matters"; this might have recontextualized our authority, our names, lives, and critical thinking all made secondary to "scientific" voices.

The editors of *Deep* represent varying subjectivities in the spectrum of SCI experience. We share genuine interests in people's stories but express this in different ways. One of us works as a research scientist and professor, her SCI a more private experience, while the other tells stories about his life following SCI for public audience, pursuing historical and legal interests related to disability and civil rights. Neither of us is a number cruncher by nature so relied more on what people tell us and what we told each other for our information. We are also significantly different, one man and one woman, one European-American and one African-American, one straight and one gay. We share these variables because we believe that our complex identities of disability significantly inform the reliability and validity of our project. As the traditional researcher declares missing data, standards of error, or other invisible factors that shape and delimit the results of analysis, so do we delimit and shape this work. We tried to make ourselves real and available to anyone with SCI who wanted to write.

We are not much removed from the people we are studying, however clear our scientific and community objectives may be. We are both analytical thinkers, trained in disciplines that favor close interrogation and argument as part of producing knowledge. For these reasons, we consider ourselves part of the group, our characteristics merged into the greater demographic of our writers.

We are five men and five women, four of whom are white/European-American descent, four of whom are African-American or Latino-American, and two of whom identify as mixed-race, including Asian- and Native-American backgrounds. Diverse in religion, class, sexual orientation, and geography, our authors all sustained disabling spinal cord injuries, although we differ as to how long ago they sustained them (from two years ago to forty-two years ago) and to what degree of injury they sustained (resulting in life-theatening complete quadriplegia to milder, incomplete paraplegia). One of us did not survive to see the publication of this volume, as we will discuss later in this introduction. The editors elected to keep our pool of writers small so as to concentrate on the project's depth, but in retrospect, we noted a surprising parallel between our author group and a portrait of diversity in our region.

Deep also tries to dislodge the popular misconception about disability that it is connected to human bodies and stays there. Marva Ways explains in her exploration of how people with SCI are perceived, "We do not need to feel stopped because we are not standard." Disability is largely a social, psychological, political and spiritual phenomenon, one whose popular idea is heavily influenced by medical and religious authority. Asking our participating authors to speak from the authority of SCI experience, as these essays show, resulted in our writing more often about times and places, relationships and contexts, politics and beliefs. Linked together as a kind of community deliberation on the themes that surround us, sometimes clearly, sometimes imperceptibly, the results of our writing assumes *some* common body experiences based on traditional medical and rehabilitation interventions, then diverges to explore tremendous difference.

We began with what we have in common and searched for what made us distinct. We started creating *Deep* in the spring of 2005 as an inclusive writing initiative about life experience after spinal cord injury, openly inviting members of the SCI community through a state wide network and newsletter produced by the Model SCI Care System at the University of Michigan, Ann Arbor. We used a "concept outline" to detail the idea of having people author on issues and themes they think about now that they live with spinal cord injuries.

Participants were asked to choose a theme that "the jury was out on", i.e., a hypothetical concept we would explore rhetorically with one eye on the subject, another on ourselves, and a "third eye" on the world. This "depth perspective" surfaces almost immediately in Charles Beatty, Jr.'s work, for example, a stereoscopic exploration of risk, now and then: "Even my riskiest act, the one I know only because the words 'spinal cord injury' tell me was really, really bad—even this act could have been worse." Working in several sessions with an editor, Beatty encounters the many-faceted phenomenon of risk in his life, having survived two SCIs.

How we came to our topics varied slightly in method, some of us starting with a clear hypothesis while others wrote toward their own concerns and named their work. Several authors have chosen themes that would launch them to talk about other complex ideas; Tom Hoatlin moves between what is remarkable and faithful, Cindy Russette shifts from inconvenience to the social politics of disability barriers in places of employment and in our homes.

We flexed our research mode by expanding the writing time, place, manner, and writing approach employed in our sessions. Authors worked on-site at the Department of Physical Medicine and Rehabilitation, at home, in nursing homes, in rehab, in cafes. Sessions varied from half an hour to four hours in length. Editors took different actions with each author, ranging from simple listening and response, typing or transcribing, interviewing, and setting words in prose, careful to preserve the "voice" of each author in content and style. Most authors wrote their essays over several months' time, a process due in part to the reflective nature of writing profoundly and also because our disabilities often altered our schedules and our energies.

Several of us experienced important self-transformation as a result of narrating our "real lives". We were able to confirm that some of what we think and feel is indeed true. Travar Pettway works through layers of necessary lies to unearth the value of honesty for society and for us as individuals. In addition, we were able to write our ways toward what we could not earlier figure out. In the language of research scientists, we wrote our ways towards self-actualization. In the language of authorship, we wrote our ways toward real lives that felt more lively and accessible. Marcy Epstein echoes this idea from the other edge of real life, mortification, in her coming-out tale as a woman humbled by a mild SCI.

In the spirit of experiment, these essays come with rough currents and rip tides, wearing down and revealing the bareness and vulnerability that many of us feel after our injuries, and also the jagged, emotional edges that conflict with a world that is just discovering that we are human beings who use chairs. Some authors express a beautiful catharsis, like Barbara Gough, who rediscovers self-worth from the shift of family obligations. Danny Heumann's essay on sex and manhood, in contrast, churns up a number of scientific and cultural frustrations in his search for amazing disability-positive sex. Marc Navarro ruminates ambivalently on reconnecting in deeper friendships after SCI. Both men write in waves of declaration and despondency, their works reflecting, respectively, one's tireless advocacy for stem cell technology and another's comeback as a head-banging song writer.

Anaïs Nin once wrote, "People living deeply have no fear of death." Nin airs the difficult difference between those of us who strike at depth and those of us who live within it. The lived-experience of SCI throws us into the spray of this problem. Some of us touch the depth of our being coolly, briefly, and others of us feel buried alive in our own molten cores. While she feared neither death nor its opposite, such deep intensity changed the course of living for Julie Harrison. Julie was one of our ten writers, a research assistant in rehabilitative psychology, a woman with spinal cord injury after a high premeditated fall, and a disability community leader who passed away on November 30, 2005.

Hard as it was for us, and we imagine for family and friends, Julie's difficulty grew in residing in two places, the lived experience of manic-depression and SCI and the figurative, sheer and sometimes unconventional sense she had of meaning. She was ill but could mask it with confidence and warmth. She finished a degree in Psychology, trained as a massage therapist. She read, wrote letters, attended talks and seminars. Julie knew the transformative power of narrative for illness and well-being.

Perhaps like many of us with SCI and other disabilities, Julie sought the completion of her plot, how her mental heroism would come out in the end. Sadly we tell too few stories in which the unwell find their ways to feeling better. She persisted for answers from the medical and psychological community for the ways she was feeling and spoke with many about how it felt not to find the right answers. Not getting sufficient answers for her was perhaps one of the most frustrating and enraging measurement of her struggle to persist in surviving. She couldn't do anything about what she couldn't pinpoint.

Without those answers, other terrible possibilities would creep in. This defined hopeless for her, her mom Sherry says. Julie was incredibly articulate about this doom, since without sufficient illumination about her health she would sit in darkness, wondering, despite all her goodness in deed and companionship, if she harbored an inexorable evil. Julie's physical disability was accepted by her. She told her mother she did not mean that her SCI was some sort of payback. If anything, Julie rocked the world from her chair.

Fish in water and woman on land, Julie traversed her personal and professional worlds in a manner that most researchers and most women would not dare. For this book she was composing an essay on the patience she had developed since acquiring her injury. Simultaneously in the fall of 2005 she was protesting aggressive policies by the Bush Administration for a group called World Can't Wait! In excitement, Julie offered to shoot our cover work for the publication, an image of herself in the favorite Halloween costume of a mermaid, diving deep into the clear expanse of an exercise pool. We have her picture but not what she saw.

In the cover work and frontispiece of Michelle Leon, who lives with physical disability in the United Kingdom, we offer an imaginary image of Julie Harrison, since she could seem mermaidenly. Leon's keen drawing of the mermaid has her do all the things we thought she couldn't do. She breaks with any expectation of her, standing on flippers, tending to schools of fish. As Julie planned to swim deep in writing, on the cover a fish-person swims about in men's heads, of all places finding a place for repose, a place to sit and be, in the matters and muds of the mind. Forget the mind-body split, the mermaid appears to say. *Live in your experience.* She tells it like it is, complete with the mythos attached to the mermaid that suggests Julie's earthiness and fluidity, beauty and intelligence, and fleetingness.

Less obvious about the figure of the mermaid for our revered friend and peer, Julie delicately balanced what she needed and what she had, reminding us that she was far from mythic. Her experience as a woman with multiple disabilities exhilarated her, but, as it is for many people suffering from severe depression and mood difficulties following disability, it sometimes made her life feel unbreathable. We trust that Julie's commitment and passion may be felt in this book, which includes one of her last writings on disability. Her work tells us that any work on people with SCI that would hold water or be worth its salt, must courageously, vigorously, and visibly depict the depth and expanse of human possibility. This book is dedicated to Julie to help her possibilities become true in other people's lifetimes.

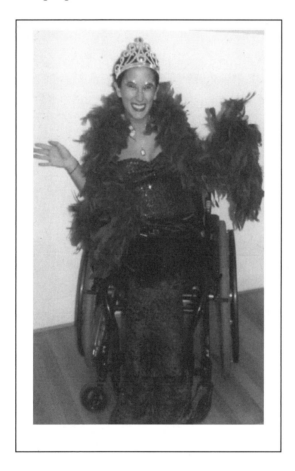

1

BARBARA GOUGH ON OBLIGATION

Let me start by telling you a little bit about myself. I am a wife, mother, grandmother, sister, and friend. I am also a newly disabled woman who is only two years into my journey of being disabled. I did not have an accident or do anything that could have caused my legs to stop working. My disability came from an infection in my cerebral spinal fluid after back surgery. It has changed my life and the lives of those who love me. It has changed many of the obligations that we all have and many of the ways we interact with each other.

Before I got ill, I worked hard to become who I was, without too much thought for the path I was taking. I married a man very different from myself when I was only 19 years old. We have been married for 39 years, and Allen has filled my life with practicality and other characteristics I am missing. He is a retired computer engineer whose job required us to move to different states. That was both a good thing and a bad thing. Moving was a good thing because it gave us the opportunity to meet and become friends with so many different kinds of people. It was a bad thing because we had to work hard to give our children a sense of knowing and belonging to an extended family of our own.

My husband and I have had a good marriage, although it is not perfect. Over the years we have had to make lots of changes. We have two children—a daughter Kimberly, who is a successful attorney and the mother of our three grand-children—and a son Allen, III, who is a successful retail manager. Both of our children are married to individuals we love and respect. Our marital struggles and successes result from the ways Allen and I divided the many responsibilities we shared. We lived traditionally, which meant that our obligations to each other were clearly defined, not by any profound communication between us, but rather by the tried and true ways that our society sets for men and women together.

I was a stay–at–home mother whose primary obligation was to take care of the family. And I did my job well. My daughter was no problem as a child, and we had a lot of fun when she was young. Funny and over-adventurous, my son was more of a challenge when he was a boy. I was always his main supporter when he was growing up. In the colorful domain of motherhood, I took any and every obligation with great seriousness. I never minded all that my son, daughter, and husband needed from me. After all, I loved them. What they could not do for themselves, I gladly did for them. This was instinct.

Do we have instincts toward our own nurturing? My obligations to myself, beside the obligations of motherhood, were a murkier picture, although I did not know it then. After my children were grown, I went back to college and finished my undergraduate and master's degrees. I had a successful job and served on the Board of Directors for my international professional association. Everything seemed to go well as I made my own way. My two grown children were both successful. My husband loved me. I enjoyed a great job, status in a professional organization, and an adjunct professorship in the academic world. I was able to make investments in our future, buy some valuable art, and purchase additional things that successful people acquire. I carried a lot in my life without fully understanding the critical weight of the load. My transformation into a woman with more profound obligations to herself and her disability arrived both abruptly and painfully when I had standard surgery for a herniated lumbar disc.

My surgery did not go well. I had headaches that would not go away. I required three surgeries in three days and they still did not correct the original problem. Then, infections in my cerebral spinal fluid required doctors to perform multiple surgeries on my brain. I was in the hospital for six months. I can't remember much of the months prior to my surgery or most of the time I was in the hospital. God has sheltered me from the pain of my illness. I do know that the outcomes from the surgeries caused many of the obligations that my family, friends, and I had to change dramatically.

I was always the caregiver in our family. I did the shopping, cleaning, raising kids, cooking, and paying the bills. Now I needed others to take care of me. The funny thing that my spinal cord injury has taught me is that to find myself, I have had to give my care over to others in a way I never have experienced safely before. This was a very difficult change for me, as well as for those who love me. Most of my life had been about supporting others. Most of my life had proceeded in ignorance of deeper debts and deeper losses. How could I just sit here and let others care for me? I felt like such a burden on those who loved me.

I feel I am alive today because of my husband's love and his marital obligations towards me. In order to survive, I at first *had to,* and now understand I *can,* rely on Allen's care. Feeling the weight of my care shift to his shoulders delivered a refreshing shock to me. Allen became my primary care-giver, my advocate, and my protector. He cared for my earliest needs after the SCI. He fed me, interacted with the doctors, shielded me from others, and made decisions about my care. It was no accident that the memories of my illness and events surrounding my six month hospitalization have been entrusted to him. I simply don't have them. I always knew Allen loved me. I just never realized the actions he would take to prove that love. And I never before understood the capacity in myself to accept that love and to honor his obligation as my husband.

This changing of roles did place a huge burden on Allen. He had to complete all of my former responsibilities as he picked up the burdens of our everyday life. Because he picked up so many and lifted such a heavy load from me, for the first time I can remember I could see that my own obligations were worthy. Not all the shifts in burden of this transition into disabled life ran one way. In his own way and time, Allen learned this as well, embracing the true meaning of being the provider he was intended to be. This lesson was not learned in an instant. During the time I was so sick, his mother passed away and he did not have the opportunity to mourn her death. He suffered with severe depression, losing his sense of worth, his job, and over 60 pounds. As I started to recover, Allen began to get worse. I became more aware of his difficulties as I got better. What I am describing to you is the importance we have found in observing the unique shape of our transformation together, the ups and downs of a marriage as I recover from this acute injury.

Allen came to the hospital every day and spent most of the day with me. As his depression worsened, he would come to visit me and stay only for a short time, explaining that he had things to do at home to get ready for my return. When my sister came from Florida to help him with me, she discovered he had not done anything. He had been so depressed that it had interfered with his doing ordinary tasks. I never confronted him on this. He told me one day that he was not even able to make it to the grocery store. I worried about him as I saw him lose so many pounds. He finally went to see a doctor to help him learn how to face his new obligations to me, to our family, and to himself. Imagine, two people realizing at the same time that our roles and our burdens of necessity had to change, could change, and would change, all for the better. This was Allen and me.

During my illness two major events took place in our family. My son, whom we call Trey, got married while I was still in the hospital. He and his bride–to–be offered to change the date of their wedding, but my husband told them not to delay their happiness on our account. Trey told me that all he wanted to do at his wedding was dance with his mom, but I told him I could not dance anymore. It was easier to jump on the first assumption I could think of rather than confront the new ways I could be in the world. People in wheelchairs don't dance, I thought, but Trey had asked me to do this for him, and I wanted this for him. I was his mom. I had only changed in my eyes, not in his. To do for him as I had always done, I needed to let others take care of me so that I could nurture my son. I could not accept less from myself and he would not accept less from me. He came to the hospital for us to practice dancing—he on his feet and me in my wheelchair.

I cried when he left because I felt inadequate as a parent and thought I was putting a terrible burden on him.

On his wedding day, I got in my gorgeous blue dress, dyed–to-match shoes, and wavy wig that my daughter bought for me and was put in my wheelchair The dress made me feel beautiful and the wig hid my shaved head. Checking me out of the hospital, my husband put me in the accessible van he had just purchased. Every time he stopped for traffic or a light, I would slide under the seat belt, a little more and more out of my wheelchair. Who would have thought that a chiffon dress would slide so much on the cushion over my seat? Allen was frightened so much that he thought something was going to happen to me. He said that we could not continue to the wedding because he was afraid--likely another sign of his depression. I was laughing at the situation while Allen was yelling at me that this was not funny. He stopped and got me back into the wheelchair; I pleaded with him to take me to the wedding. When we got to the reception hall, Trey and his best man had to reseat me so I could attend the festivities. With Allen so tense, it was all he could do to sit rigidly nearby.

When the time came for our dance, Trey took my hand in his and led me to the floor in my wheelchair. I was so happy and proud of him. I was afraid that I would cry but we both had smiles on our faces during our time together. When it was over, I looked at my family and other guests who were all standing, watching us, and crying. Even in my wheelchair, we had had our special moment. Trey was far more perceptive than I because he realized how important his obligations to his mother were. From that moment, I realized how the obligations of my role as the caregiver of the family had continued but changed.

At the same time in my illness that plans for Trey's wedding were under way, my daughter Kimberly, who was pregnant with triplets, sadly lost one of her babies. One of my few memories during this time was of Kimberly crying very quietly at my bedside and telling me that one of her babies would be stillborn. She could see what I could not see—that I was not capable then of sharing her loss, of feeling the sadness, the upset for her I feel so much now. This, I learned from my medical team, was natural, since my body could only handle just what it needed to heal.

Kimberly's twin girls were born almost eight weeks early, small but healthy. I was able to leave my hospital to see my daughter and her wonderful new daughters at their hospital. My feelings have since returned. I wish now that I had been able to put my arms around Kimberly and let her cry. I will always feel it was her worry and concern for me that caused her loss.

As the eldest, Kimberly took on my role as family caregiver. I believe this placed a big burden on her because she had to manage more of our family's activities. Together with my loving son–in–law, she spent a lot of time at the hospital sitting with her father and me helping make decisions pertaining to my care and providing support for her father. When I came home from the hospital, she cooked family Sunday dinners. Where once I would have taken over her responsibilities, she took over many of mine. She told me she was taking on my role and its obligations just for a little while until I was well enough to handle them again. Because of my new disability she had to reach into her motherhood even deeper, deep enough for both of us. She says that sometimes she'd like to be a child again and learn from me, her mother.

Although I didn't know it at the time, my four sisters, brother, and sister-in-law, in their concern for me, left their own families to come to be with me. This was surprising, since I am the eldest and not used to the idea that all of them would and could care for my family and me. Since my injury, I have observed that our families can actually change and our comfort zones expand in overlapping ways that make us all close and more appreciative of each other. I have few memories of them being with me in the intensive care unit, but each has shared their recollections of that time with me. They all took on some of my obligations as the "oldest" sibling in the family.

After I had been home from the hospital for awhile, my sisters all came for a "sister's week-end." It was truly love and a found sense of obligation that brought them to Michigan in January from Florida, Arizona, and New York. I was anxious for them to see that with a lot of practice, I could again do for myself some of the tasks I used to do, which was a big accomplishment for me. I always knew my sisters and brother loved me, I just did not know that they could inspire and help me. They provided me with love and a closeness that I can't describe because they could be there for my family and me when we needed them. They tell me I am an inspiration for them, not because I am disabled but because I am learning and growing again to the best of my ability. And I can let myself feel their love. That love and support is far more significant than the material signs of success that I once thought so important.

I would be remiss if I did not touch on the special role of friends in giving me their love and support. Friends were my "gifts from God." More importantly, friends provided a unique element: they volunteered because they wanted to, not because they were obligated to me like family. My friends, always an important part of my life, grew closer during and after my illness. They could exercise choices among their obligations while I benefited by knowing they chose to keep and deepen our connections. I often think of my best friend

Penny, who comes from 30 miles away to encourage me when my sense of self-obligation slips, or who gets me going when I would rather not. Penny is not scared of my wheelchair. She just loves me. She chooses me and she chooses my life with my injury. She and other friends supported Allen and my children during their time of need. They would tell me they knew I was strong enough to survive, and stretched themselves even further to worry about Allen or provide comfort for our children when I could not. Penny and others were obliged to me rather than obligated, but they took on the very spirit of obligation. My friends' obligations to me had changed how I view options in our care for one another.

But has my spinal cord injury changed me? Not at all, for I am still me. My injury helped me realize I made a contribution to this world and that I mattered. My illness shifted the balance between me and many family members--most of all with my husband. I learned I mattered most to him.

When sudden shifts in what we owe each other occur, both husbands and wives will typically experience much stress. In the beginning, I was fearful that I had lost my

identity as the good wife, while Allen feared some new catas-
trophe. He labored somewhat pessimistically under his new
burden of attending to my care at home. When I came home
from the hospital he was even afraid to sleep in the same bed
with me. He thought he would break me, something we were
both afraid to discuss with each other but which hung over us
like a dead weight. With many of the mistakes we made, our
confidence grew because we learned I would not break under
his touch. Additionally, Allen learned that he could handle
me in most circumstances with great success. When he came
back to our bed to sleep with me it was a wondrous sign of his
acceptance of new roles for us and the beginning of the end of
his depression. For me it marked the beginning of my self-
acceptance, not only as a wife, but as a person of special
worth, worthy of a strengthened marital bond.

Part of my thinking about what we owe each other as
trusted mates, regardless of spinal cord injury, concerns our
sex life. I worried about how things would be between us
even when I was in the hospital. Allen and I have always had
an active sex life, one that had been an important part of our

relationship. This was often the way we used to make up after a disagreement. I had to face the reality that our sex life needed to change or it could become a real burden in our marriage. Allen had to accept different ways for me to satisfy his needs so that he would know I wanted and needed him. Although I can no longer "feel" the sensuality of traditional sex, I definitely "feel" the closeness of our love and enjoy our bodies together. I have found new meaning in being kissed and held. Now, I have become more at peace with my body and with how my own sexual needs are met. There is something often left unspoken in our quest for a normal sex life that I think is truly important. My body's simplest sexuality is its own aliveness, the awareness I have come to after my spinal cord injury that my body is mine and something worth my care and my desire.

Besides being unable to perform some of the activities I thought important as a wife and mother, I also lost the career that was so symbolic to me. I had worked so hard for my career and was dismayed to see it go. I can no longer work at what I used to do because I cannot think like I used to. I thought I had to give up the many things that my work allowed us to have. However, I have learned that the things I once thought were important do not matter much at all.

Sorting through these things was tough because it was not clear how I felt about things. For example, we had a big, beautiful home that was no longer accessible to me. It had four levels, but I only had access to one level, the family room and an office that had been converted into a bedroom for me. At first I thought I had burdened my husband because we had to sell our home and buy a new one that gave me more accessibility. But our new home is better for both of us and has given us something new to work on together. I also gave up my new Cadillac STS (which I loved and felt so suave driving) for an accessible Chrysler minivan. The car was one of those things that I considered a symbol of my success. I learned, however, that the kind of car you drive just does not matter as long as it gets you where you want to go. The minivan does just that. And we are good to ourselves in caring about where and how we go forward.

⁘

One of the hardest things I have had to rethink after my SCI was our vision of retirement. Allen and I used to play golf together and belonged to a local country club. We had plans to retire to a golfing community in Tennessee, spending part of our time on the golf course and part of it back in Michigan with our children and grandchildren. We owned a piece of property on a golf course but one of the first things Allen did when I got sick was to sell the property. Along with that sale we lost our retirement dreams, and dreams are the hardest things to replace. Most of us struggle just to make each day flow together smoothly, with dreams of retirement a far off goal. Now my husband had a wife who could not golf with him to the end of our days. But he never gave up on me. He consistently made me feel like I mattered to him and reassured me that we would find new things to do together. Turns out we may play golf together after all, with some adaptation, of course.

Allen and I have taken on the challenge of finding

new dreams. We both like to travel and we have taken several small trips in Michigan. We just completed a three-week driving trip of the southern United States during which we even attended a golf match together. The trips around Michigan were no problem; however, the trip to the South presented more challenges and learning opportunities. Since the enforcement of the Americans with Disabilities Act, this country is becoming more and more accessible, with some places more so than others. We also discovered we did not have to sacrifice seeing or doing much to enjoy being in a new place. Most important, we learned that we both must have patience when dealing with my care. We have a vacation planned where we will be flying. When I was working, I used to fly all over the world. This will be my first flying trip with a spinal cord injury and I am a little nervous about it. But I have learned that I have the courage to face that challenge, and I will.

As we go on with our injuries, our responsibilities don't change. My experiences have taught me that everyday incidents can become milestones for growth and opportunities to assert myself. For example, one day I ran away from home. Allen and I had had a little fight. After we got home from shopping, he left me locked in my wheelchair down in the van while he took groceries into the house. Then he unlocked the wheelchair and left me to get out of the van by myself. I knew I could get out by myself, but Allen had always stayed to close the door after me. This time he did not. I was really ticked and decided to run away. I left our house and the neighborhood, crossed a busy divided four–lane highway, went into another neighborhood, and headed by sidewalk to my daughter's home. In my travels I hit a few areas that did not have sidewalks so had to travel on a busy highway. I got stuck in some gravel and two strangers stopped to help me get out. I was determined to reach my daughter's home, side-walks or no sidewalks.

Back at our house, when I did not come in, Allen went out to look for me, only to discover me long gone. He looked around the yard and then drove through the neighborhood trying to find me. When he could not, he called 9–1–1. Bloomfield Township police came out, looked around our home for me, and questioned Allen closely to determine if he had done something to me before they sent others out to find me. After two hours, they called neighboring police agencies and fire departments to help in the search for an adult woman in a wheelchair who had simply decided to take matters into her own hands.

Four miles from home, I was zooming along Middle-belt Road when a policeman stopped me to ask where I was going. I told the police officer that I was angry with my husband and I was going to my daughter's house. He was very kind to me now that the emergency was over. He called to tell others where he had found me, and they notified Allen. By the time my husband arrived, four policemen in four cars were waiting in line behind me as the traffic whizzed by. The men just smiled at me when I got into our van and told me I should not go off by myself again. I told them I was glad to have given them something to do on a Sunday morning. I smiled to myself that I was going to do exactly what I wanted, a notion that was a far cry from the traditional housewife I once had been. All Allen said to me after giving me a big tearful hug and seeing that I was okay, was, "Next time take your cell phone with you so I can at least make sure you are all right."

We never had words over what I did, and I simply can't explain how independent I felt. I had the best time I had had in a long time. I was free and in charge again. I had a new sense that I could take care of myself and I felt so proud. I looked at the beautiful homes and gardens I passed with different eyes. I appreciated everything I did in a different way. I knew I could be successful on my own--a very good discovery for me. My sense of being a burden on others had lessened and my sense of my obligation to myself was renewed.

Allen and I both have transformed our obligations to each other after to my injury, which I believe has added new meaning to our lives. I have realized a total shift in my thinking, actions, and beliefs. The things that were important to me before I got sick are not as important to me now. Although I have always loved my husband, I have found a new love and appreciation for him as he encourages me to try old, new, or different things. Different as we are, we have learned to value the strengths we each bring to our marriage and the weight we pull.

Allen has always seen the glass as half empty while I have seen the glass as half full. Our natural obligations to each other have given us a strong marriage that has equaled one whole glass. Sometimes I ask him still if I am a huge burden to him and he tells me no. We know though, that in truth, we are burdens to each other. The difference is that after my spinal cord injury, we are both aware that if we want our marriage and our lives for ourselves to be all that they can be, we need to allow each other to express ourselves in new and vibrant ways. I believe that our experiences have enlightened both of us and have strengthened the ties that bind us.

I have a long way to go in my recovery and further still to go in my exploration of myself in this world. I have been given an opportunity for a richer life. Every day I feel I can accomplish more than I did yesterday. I am learning to cook again, to do the laundry, and am taking over more of my former household chores. Although these are things I used to do with ease, they now feel new to me. Things take longer and sometimes need to be done in different ways. I care for myself more and more, each day trying to do new and different things physically, emotionally, and intellectually. I know that the future holds many new obligations for me to face. Although my responsibilities have become more challenging, they are not really more burdensome and I am no less obligated to meet them.

I don't like the terms "handicapped" or "disabled." To me these paint a negative picture of a person who can't do anything or who desires less. I know I am different than I used to be. I can't walk. I can't feel things waist down. I can't hear out of one ear. I have to think more deliberately than I used to and must work harder for my brain to function. But I get better every day. I am only two years into my recovery and am already finding ways to make my life even more meaningful and less cumbersome (I don't mean this just physically) both to those who love me and to myself.

Being disabled is not the end of life but rather a new and different beginning. It unquestionably changes your obligations as well as the obligations of those around you. Attitude has a lot to do with success. Most of the time, I stay positive and tuned in to the critical issues, and this takes me through the rough patches. When my attitude is not right, I now turn openly to family and friends to put me back on the right track. They give me more reasons to be happy and well. They remind me of the greater debt I owe to the fact that I am alive, I am injured, and I am still deeply loved.

My hope is that after reading my story that you, the reader, will find the courage you need to take small steps to meet the challenges and obligations of your life. They won't be easy steps to take, but with the right attitude and mind-set you can accomplish them. Keep in mind that the world is not yet easily accessible for people with disabilities. Some people balk at their obligations while others think those of us with disabilities are burdens. However, there are countless people who do not look at us as burdens and millions of things you can do to carry your own weight. I embrace the choices I have now in the obligations I wish to carry into my future. My hope is that you, the reader, will find great healing and growth by accepting support from family and friends and choosing the obligations you wish to embrace. The great strength and love you may receive from others can lead to other unexpected successes in life after spinal cord injury, and you may find yourself even more obligated to those important people or more importantly, to yourself.

2

Sometimes I wonder what people see of me when I go out. Is it some fictitious character or façade construed from the looks of my equipment? Is it what I want them to see? What do I want them to see? Do I want them to see my intelligence? Do I want them to see strength? Or do I want them to see someone who has needs and doesn't move his arms and legs? When I really think about it, I want people to see all of these things. But are they contradictory? How can I be strong yet be in need? How can I be intellectually fit yet "handicapped"? Beyond these contradictions of what is the

27

honest truth about me is another important truth, one that appears questionable and dishonest. Honestly, what we all want people to see is whatever would be beneficial to us at that time.

With that said, is our projection from ourselves as persons with disabilities beneficial to us or a problem? Is it okay to manipulate people, institutions, etc., toward these projections? The reason I pose all these questions is because when I need assistance from our government or my insurance companies, I am perceived as a needy, semi-helpless case. This transaction over my identity starts me wondering: how does this influence government policy toward me? How does it influence the decisions that my medical insurers make? Does my appearance, honest or not, make government policy of giving me just the things I need to sustain myself but not enough to advance myself fair? What if the terms of my transaction were to change? For instance, if I were to get a job and pay taxes, I would lose my health insurance. Does that seem right to you? Wouldn't it be more feasible to allow me some type of supplemental health care for my spinal cord injury while I work and contribute back to the state by paying taxes? Wouldn't that require them to see me as independent and needy at the same time?

My point is that if I were completely honest with the government, then I would let them see that I am an intelligent, capable, and ambitious human being instead of trying to convince them that I am a "vent-dependent quadriplegic" not at all capable of providing for myself. If I were completely honest, I would show my insurance company that I do not always need what they give me. But I accept their allocations for fear that if I don't, they will take too much back in their effort to be less wasteful. To illustrate, I receive thirty tracheotomy care kits every month when all I really need is the brush inside of each kit. But they won't allow me to get the brush alone. I have not pushed the issue for fear that they might determine that other things I really do need, like catheters or gloves, are also less necessary. So if I were completely honest, I would show them that I am an intelligent individual who is capable of managing my care and whatever supplies I get allotted with a lot more frugality and efficiency than they can. But I don't.

Similarly, if I were completely honest with my family, I would show them a Travar who at times gets depressed, lonely, and even angry. Instead I am always Travar the Strong or Travar the Superman. I never let people into that part of my life. Many of us don't let people into those parts of our lives for fear of judgment. Speaking of honesty, and honestly speaking, is this fair? We pretend that family ties are held together by unconditional love, but it seems that many times there are conditions that go unspoken.

Tell me this: what type of relationship do you feel you can have with an uncle, brother, or cousin who gets depressed, lonely, and angry? By any means, I am not saying that you can't and won't love someone like that. But won't there be certain conditions? For instance, if your relative is constantly depressed, couldn't that wear out your own happiness to a significant degree? Likely you would not want to be around him as often. If that person always felt lonely, despite trying your best to help him out of a rut, wouldn't you eventually stop reaching out as much? And if that person were often angry, wouldn't you try to avoid being the target of that anger? So in order for you to have a relationship with this person, the conditions would be, "I can't deal with you when you are depressed . . . angry . . . too pained from loneliness. And I won't help you if you don't help yourself."

Ideally this kin of yours would be allowed the whole range of his emotions, positive and negative. Personally, I would like to function for a day as I really am without that being understood as my having some sort of condition, problem, or crisis. If I were completely honest, I would let my family see a Travar who doesn't always want to get out of bed, I would let them see a bummed-out Travar and hope that they would still see Travar the Human Being. I would let them see a Travar who gets upset when I think about the circumstances of my injury. If I were completely honest, I would let them see the whole Travar.

What is it about our power, our psyches, that seems always to pass initial judgment on who people are? Right or wrong, why do we always try to figure a person out based on very little information, such as looks or how well they communicate? What does having a spinal cord injury really tell people? Ultimately our perceptions of people are usually based on our own preconceived notions, and that is what we present as people who are disabled. This presentation is what we have to do in order to survive. Why can't we as disabled people be seen as what we are? We all have different injuries or sicknesses, different personalities, different capabilities, but at the end of the day, we are all just *disabled*. In *all* honesty, we are just *ourselves*.

Woven into our society is a certain strain of tolerance for dishonesty when it comes to our public selves as people with disabilities. This is not because we are special in any way, but since most people conduct themselves differently among others in order to achieve social benefits, we pretty much follow suit. To pick and choose our public and private selves is usually normal. What is normal for the mainstream, however, is not allowed to be normal for us. What is normal for us, from the point of view of the outside, is only our dependence, complacency, and underachievement with little pressure to succeed. We are framed with this dishonesty. For example, do you think you would ever hear the parent of a disabled kid say that when she is eighteen she needs to get a job or move out of the house?

Before my injury, I was just a seventeen-year-old Black male who really did not stand out and could have been easily perceived as a guy who would snatch your purse. I wore my pants hanging off my butt and every word out of my mouth was slang. I hung out with rough kids and fought a lot, and despite being around a lot of stuff, never did much criminally beside brawl at school and ride around unknowingly in a stolen car. I was seen as just another dumb kid who would not get far.

After being caught in violent crossfire and sustaining my SCI, all of a sudden I became intelligent to some people. I have no brain damage, so my personality has not changed. I am still the same person, but now, eleven years later, I am embraced as someone with potential, an all-around good guy. I still live in the same skin. I still have the same frame of mind and the same pants. If you were to be completely honest with yourself, you would admit that seeing a six-foot-one Black male standing up gives you a different feeling than the same man sitting in a wheelchair, despite him being the *same person*. Even other Black people react to me differently. The contrast is there. I simply seem less threatening now that I have been shot in the neck.

So where then does my injury leave me in the eyes of others and in my own? Am I a burden? No! Should I just subsist or should I be left to just exist? No! Should I have to have to be strong every day? No! I should be accepted as *Travar*! You should be accepted as *you*! We cannot and should not be reduced to the connotations of our spinal injuries!

Must we change to fit either the negative or positive ideals of disability? Shouldn't these representations of us change instead? Imagine yourself as a person with a spinal cord injury who *exceeds* every low expectation. Imagine a world where companies heavily recruited people with disabilities for the sake of diversity and gave us all the benefits we needed plus seven "I don't want to get out of bed days" each year. Imagine a world where people with disabilities are the people who get to set our own legislative agenda and assume more responsibility in the solutions to disability-related problems. If we fully lived in this world today, wouldn't we have a more honest dialogue about who we are, what we need, and what we want? Yes! Could we not just be ourselves, without the appearances and the assumptions? Now I wouldn't put some guy in a wheelchair into a particular role *just because*. Honestly, some people in wheelchairs can be creeps. Then again, so are some of our non-disabled politicians. But put some civic-minded people like us in state and federal government, and the dialogue becomes more fluid between the people who pose honest problems and the people who find honest solutions.

I am criticizing but not judging those with disabilities, for we have the primary and difficult responsibility in showing an honest picture of who and what we are. At the moment, disability stereotypes are a hindrance, another set of barriers we need to build ramps over. If we are committed to removing the barriers between the perceptions of society and our wholeness as people with spinal cord injuries, we require a third sort of honesty beyond individual and social honesty about people with disabilities.

This third honesty reflects a shift away from tolerating dishonesty about ourselves as disabled people and toward tolerating more honesty about how disability *works* within the culture that both the individual and society comprise. Honestly, we are not in a good place right now. Right now we are in a subservient place, an infantile state in which we are just getting to know ourselves and our world is just beginning to recognize us. On one hand I see the growth of disability studies while on the other I see the erosion of the ADA in the higher courts. We are being led through this life by the hand.

What is the hand that leads us? In our personal lives, the hand is what our culture deals us, the overall impression that our spinal cord injuries mean most significantly how we now *compare* in relationship to non-disabled people, their bodies, and their being. In truth, we can be and are compared, but this culture of "normalcy" misses the intense significance of our *difference*. We cannot be compared! Honestly, the measurement of our being is not the norm but our "deviation" from those norms. We're different! The measuring stick needs to be turned around. Let us lead our world by our hands, our atrophic hands, our still hands, our powerful hands. Our hands in leading this world toward more tolerance of honesty depend upon our differences in disability. Our hands may sit still but there is latent power waiting to be released. We maintain an integral physical relationship with the universe, and it is up to those of us who can speak to the power of our difference to make this known.

Difference is not such a bad thing. My injury was a blessing because it brought my life into perspective, when I may not have gained otherwise. My wheelchair has led me to places that my legs could never have taken me; to the University of Michigan and to unforeseen desires for a future beyond a crime-riddled neighborhood. I learn my strengths and weaknesses now, in part because there is so much to know about myself as a man with a spinal cord injury. I made my transition from boyhood to manhood in this chair. I have helped raise kids from my wheelchair. Beyond the comparison they could easily have made between me and a father who controls his own limbs, they have learned that no love is lost in my disability. I respect my *difference*. They see from my example that men and women with injuries like mine are skilled people with considerable abilities.

So, if I were to be utterly and completely honest, I would venture this comment about all of us who have had spinal cord injuries: that our best honesty is not always the honesty that seems convenient or easiest for us at the time. In spite of the immediate necessity of comparing ourselves to the ideals of others about our disabilities, this dishonesty is certainly less beneficial than being ourselves, since beyond policies and perceptions, we still have our mortal lives to live. Being honest about myself is one of the indisputable powers I have as an individual. Promoting this honesty alongside society's better understanding of us is our task.

3

CYNTHIA RUSSETTE ON INCONVENIENCE

The warm summer breeze brushes my skin as I rollerblade along the quiet, tree-lined asphalt paths at our community park. I feel such an uninhibited sense of freedom and exhilaration as I skate forward, backward, and spin around. I want to continue on forever. Free from the constraint of the waking world, I watch mothers push their babies in strollers and contemplate what's next. Horseback riding, tennis, waterskiing—anything in this great outdoors is mine, now and in the moments to follow. I hold on to this freedom that carries me forward, releasing and boosting me through a delicious visitation between my past and my future.

The alarm rings for the fourth time, finally waking my husband and me. The summer morning sun indeed shines through the window bright and clear, bringing another beautiful weekend day. I stretch, letting the sun caress my body as I lie there planning out my day. As I roll over, waking reality returns slowly, allowing me to savor the most freeing dream I remember ever having. Next to my bed are not the roller blades of the park but another set of wheels: the wheelchair I fondly call my Stupid Piece of Crap. That's okay, I am not surprised. I have used a wheelchair for thirty eight years.

After my husband helps me out of bed, I head down to the kitchen for hot coffee, rolls, and *The Detroit News*, rolling on toward a new day, *almost*. One would think that after such a long time the first inconvenience of the day wouldn't register much to me anymore; "inconvenience" could be my middle name. My chair, as we will refer to the Stupid Piece of Crap from now on, just doesn't seem to want to go where I want it to go. Upon further observation we notice that the tire on the right side is completely flat. My tires are pneumatic, so they require a certain air pressure to maintain their optimum efficiency. Losing the air out of the tire was just the first practical inconvenience of the day, nothing major. My husband Tom and I have traveled these days together for thirty years with myself piloting the wheelchair and my able-bodied mate as its co-pilot. We have become used to inconvenience as a significant part of our lives. Most days it pays to have a very good disposition and a sense of humor. We both do.

Fortunately, my husband is also talented and can fix almost anything. We head to the garage where there is another important and necessary part of our life, the air compressor. Just put in some air and be good to go. Right? Wrong! The tube has a hole in it and needs to be replaced. Easy enough. Wrong again! We have no tube.

Now common sense would dictate that after thirty years these minor crap accessories would be kept on hand and well stocked. I guess living dangerously is part of our lifestyle. On to Plan B, for basement. After thirty years of cohabitation, Tom and I have a basement strangely full of old wheelchairs and their parts. Thank heavens for a man who doesn't like to throw away things. As my husband descends to the basement to retrieve said tube from an earlier chair model, I wait "patiently". Patience is my second middle name. Patience means sitting in one place praying to Saint Anthony constantly for the miracle of finding needed things. Saint Anthony is on our side. Coming up the stairs smiling with said tube in hand, my husband again manages to avert the challenge, not letting inconvenience grow into a problem, since most wheelchair parts stores are closed weekends. Memo to self: order extra tubes.

We all have encountered at least one moment in our lives that was inconvenient; the doctor appointment that took much longer than anticipated, the bus we missed going to work, or the spice we needed running out for that special recipe we are supposed to take to friends for dinner that night. How about that flat tire on the highway on your way to your child's wedding or the sale item for which you made that special trip twenty miles one way to find they were all out and gave no rain checks? These are inconvenient aspects of life, whether minor or major. I do not remember exactly when the term inconvenient became a permanent part of my vocabulary, but it certainly has gained some importance now that I live with spinal cord injury.

The able-bodied world uses "inconvenience" as an excuse, either for not doing things that we need to do, or for avoiding the things that we must do. It is thought in this world that we can actually do something to solve our own difficulties. I don't have this sort of personality, but having had some serious inconvenience in my life after spinal cord injury, I have grown more observant on my own excuses as well as how deeply the idea of inconvenience affects my life as a woman with an SCI.

In the disabled world, inconveniences are frustrating incidents more like challenges that *must* be met. Each inconvenience for people with spinal cord injuries truly is an obstacle to the progress of our everyday lives. We simply choose to soften the meaning of those barriers for a number of reasons. We want to assert our equality and independence, for we wish to be the masterminds of the problem-solving needed in order for the barrier to be overcome. We want to spare other people's feelings. Sometimes we wish to spare ourselves. This process of owning inconvenience is a real learning experience, tough but something not to be afraid of. Instead it is an opportunity to hold close to ourselves as a source of self-acclimation and positive power in an inconvenient world.

Inconvenience has several levels of meaning. It can serve as a euphemism for true difficulty. On a deeper level, inconvenience makes us think about what we think is worth our time and energy and so draws the line between what we feel willing to do or willing to put up with versus what we feel unwilling to do or not do. Deeper still, inconvenience has social and physical meanings that demand that we look at our lives as people with disabilities in inconvenient but truthful ways. Originally I titled this essay "An Inconvenient Life" for this very reason. I did not want anyone reading this to continue thinking, for another second, that they themselves were inconvenient. Whatever level we understand inconvenience in our lives and those lives our lives affect, we can reckon with the physical, emotional, intellectual, and spiritual changes in a real and purposeful way, not just leading lives consisting of millions of inconveniences for ourselves and for others. My life has taken this other road.

The opposite of inconvenience is not necessarily *convenience*. Inconvenience exists at the edge of normal life. It sits at the periphery of our thoughts. We don't think of convenience although we look for it all the time. Whereas a sports injury like a sprained ankle is a serious inconvenience for a team, putting it out of its convenient win, traumatic spinal cord injury sits at the other end of the bench. Inconvenience is the opposite of life-threatening injuries like mine. Inconvenience lacks urgency.

I learned this the hard way, since many years ago I exchanged a childhood of convenience for a childhood of tremendous urgency. Nearly four decades ago, my life was zooming along much like any other senior in high school in 1968, for shortly I would be moving on to the next phase of my adulthood. You can imagine: the last year of high school is such an important time, one of the many milestones we strive to achieve. I had lettered in three sports, had lots of popular friends, a boyfriend who was the captain of the football and wrestling teams, and I was going away to college.

A massive understatement would be that getting an SCI was inconvenient to my girlhood self. I had my life pretty much planned out full steam ahead. I would attain a physical education degree and teach high school physical education. Second semester of my senior year was so busy. I was caught up in it all. I had completed all my necessary credits for graduation, except my economics course, so classes were a breeze. College applications had been sent and I anxiously waited to hear if I had been accepted. I was looking forward to going to Central Michigan University and living away from home on my own. There was senior prom, Senior Skip Day, and precious time with friends going in different directions in just a few months. It was all scary but since it was the natural order of how life should go, we took it all in stride.

In the last moments of that carefree yet purpose-driven time, I was injured on a trampoline while practicing for a local gymnastics meet in Livonia, Michigan. Having worked on my routine for several days, this time I would put the finishing touches on it. All was going well (how convenient!) when next I remember lying on the concrete and tile floor looking up at a clock on the wall. It was 1:23 p.m., the last minute uninterrupted by the rest of my life. I was not aware of what had actually happened or of the minutes that followed. I remember a ride in an ambulance, hospital staff telling me they were cutting off my new leotard and my objecting to this, since I knew I was going to need it for the meet the following Tuesday. (How inconvenient!) I needed to get up and go home. (I had things to do!) Of course, headstrong young woman that I was, I had no concept that the things I needed to do were to hang on and watch others save my life.

The contrast between what I experienced in the throes of my injury and what I thought about was stark. Though my friend's brother was a quadriplegic and my cousin was struck with polio, I was clueless about the world with disability in it.

In my teenager mind, disabilities happened to everybody else, and they were minor dents in the more important metal of a life blessed with possibilities and forward motion.

While a doctor pulled my neck and noisily drilled holes into the sides of my head, I thought of nothing really, my psyche unable to process this intervention as some-thing of profound importance. On a Striker frame in traction, with sixty pounds of weight hanging from tongs attached to my head, I floated between ideas of what should be happening and what was happening. My view of the room was either the ceiling or the floor. Up or down, I would forget the contraption below me and begin planning my return strategy.

In the months that followed, I made a terribly difficult transition from the life I had expected and the only path I had ever known, into a questionable future with fewer answers. The seriousness of my injury forced the things that had once felt dire in my life to be converted into something else. All of a sudden, the things I thought I must have for senior year to be complete were all conveniences. This is a heavy lesson to learn as a light-hearted teenager, where most of your world already feels like it is all dire consequence. The accident caused a C6-C7 spinal cord fracture, leaving me a quadriplegic, all four of my limbs unstably affected. At seventeen, I had no use of my legs and limited use and strength of my upper body. No prom. No Senior Skip Day. No parties. No lazy days signing yearbooks. I wasn't getting a summer job as a lifeguard, my soft, athletic body soaking up the sun. I was not going to CMU. It would be an amazing accomplishment to attend my own graduation.

It is easy to imagine what sort of loss this was, but the shift in priorities was the hardest for me to grasp. Starting another life made no sense when I was just getting around to mine. In my effort to normalize things, I wanted a diploma in my hand and the happy-go-luckiness of my friends. Like a lot of the pre-barrier-free world in those days, the brand new auditorium was not wheelchair-accessible. With assistance I was lifted up the steps and my father escorted me across the stage. My first outing since my accident, I did not expect this world to feel alien to me. But a leaden shift had already happened and that day I sat among a world of people who could no longer relate to me or make eye contact. I was a disabled girl rather than the Cindy they had always known and stuck by. Turned emotionally inside out, I saw myself as they saw me: a complication, an Other, an inconvenience in what otherwise would be their perfectly happy day.

I could not even imagine the pain and heartbreak my parents felt or what their first thoughts were when they first saw me after surgery. There was their beautiful, gregarious, outgoing daughter unable to move, feed herself, dress herself or go to the bathroom by herself. To a degree, I think we were all sure this was just going to be a temporary setback, a short period of urgency that could be converted back to convenience. Of course I would get well and walk again.

That ours would be a life redefined with inconveniences only came to us the evening my father and brothers first lifted me up the front porch steps. I realized, as they did, that I had lost my independence. Ready to fly from the nest and move toward a planned future, I could no longer freely come and go from my home. Although I was only home for one night, fear overcame my family in silent questions: what if we drop her? How will we care for her medical needs? Will society be able to accept and accommodate her? Will the world label her as too inconvenient to include? What will her future now hold? My parents installed a ramp to the front porch but I was still a prisoner in my own home because I was unable to use the ramp independently. At this point the truth of my disability came with the knowledge that independence stood at the forefront of inconvenience. So independence became our goal.

From that very moment my life was no longer a matter of convenience. In the sixties, less technology and less social and physical support was available for families of people with spinal cord injuries. Since our guidance from physical therapists and other paraprofessionals was extremely basic, often we improvised to get past major obstacles. This took more ingenuity than we could know. My mother had this, so the inconvenience of my early days was played out like a movie special, one act at a time.

I know God has a plan for all of us. Was this a cruel

joke on my parents, my brothers, and me? To have all our lives turned upside down in a split second? How would we handle the emotional, physical, and financial pain to come? My parents were looking forward to their oldest child moving on. They say God does not give us more challenges than we can handle but in this case we sure thought He was wrong. How would we ever overcome so many obstacles placed before us? My parents began to realize how my accident would have a broader impact on their lives. In their shock they were still mature and compassionate enough never to belittle our crisis, even if their daughter had changed drastically.

I withdrew because I was not who I wanted to be either. This was my initiation into a world where I no longer fit. I was no longer convenient to it. The world was no longer convenient for me. I had become the square peg who did not fit the round hole. My high school friends came and went. Fortunately, my family never waited on their own convenience to help me to free myself from the alienation of my spinal cord injury and to become a whole person again. I grew up in a traditional, Baby Boomer Catholic family. My parents were not rich, yet we never seemed to lack for anything. Mostly of solid Polish decent, we were definitely strong-willed and bull-headed. Families like ours love you no matter what. With validation and bullishness they helped me turn things around so that I was looking at my life in the face.

The winter after my accident we moved to a ranch home. My parents took on the financial responsibility of building a family room between the end of the house and garage so I could come and go as I pleased. Everything was level, both physically and figuratively, with few formal barriers. The bathroom sported a new high "handicap toilet" that was level with my wheelchair and made transferring something I could do independently. People I meet today with more recent injuries share with me how their rehabilitation taught them to be "handicapped". My family taught me how to take challenges head on, to surmount obstacles. With them, I felt love and commitment, the antidotes to alienation and self-denial. The accessibility of my home became an interesting parallel in my mind to how we emotionally handled my SCI. Physical accessibility meant accessing the unconditional coming and going of their young adult, disabled daughter. That feels like love to me to this day.

If not for other people to compare ourselves to, we would never know how good or bad we have it, and therefore how convenient or inconvenient our lives really are. As much as it is important to contrast our experiences with SCI with the experiences of those without SCI, it is crucial for us to learn from each other as people with disabilities. Perhaps in one of His most gracious acts of making an inconvenient life convenient again, God gave me my friend, Patti. After two months in the hospital, on another warm, beautiful sunny day in the beginning of May, I was transferred to a rehabilitation facility in Detroit. Until this point no one had told me I was disabled, and remember, I viewed the whole affair as a temporary gap in what would be again a flawless future. I had very little strength in my arms and hands, so physical and occupational therapy were large parts of my daily routine. Activities of Daily Living (ADL) taught me how to transfer, get dressed, maintain a bowel program, eat, and put on makeup. I might have been a quad, but eating and putting on lipstick were things for which I was well suited. After a week there, Patti arrived as my new roommate. She was a senior, too, who had broken her back in a car accident coming home from church. She had upper body strength and was paralyzed from the waist down. What she could do—grasp things well and transfer easily—I could not. What I could do—experience sensation and control my toilet habits—she could not. Our losses complemented each other. Our abilities complemented each other. We still joke that both of our good body parts make one good working woman. I suppose the other parts of us make one wild and crazy disabled woman! God knew we would need each other.

Two teenagers with spinal cord injuries can make up a tiny world, a world Patti and I defined for ourselves. We were always there for each other, with me as the leader of the gang and Patti close on my heels. At my any mention of "I have an idea," she would comically wince, "Oh, no! What now?" The twists and turns of our physical therapies together, the intense and difficult emotions we shared over our wrecked adolescence, the nitty-gritty of taking care of each other: Patti and I went through it side by side. This doesn't contradict my description of the world that turned its back on me, so I thought. Patti and I worked hard, and toward the end of July she got the news she was going home for good. I was ready to leave, too, but my doctor told me to wait for just a while longer. I cried for three days, making myself sick until finally he let me go home the same day.

I needed to be together with someone from my own generation who also had an SCI, someone who knew the difference between convenience and inconvenience in this special way. It didn't matter if we handled it well. Together we would face how inconvenient this world in which we lived was. Patti lived in Royal Oak, and I lived in Livonia. Neither of us could drive so had to rely on others to take us places. Since we both drove before our unfortunate events, this felt very inconvenient. The list of complaints about what we could and could not do was lengthy, but thanks to having each other as "sisters" in SCI, our troubles and woes felt somewhat like the list of ordinary teenagers.

At this point, my discussion of inconvenience takes two turns. On one hand, Patti and I ganged up and fought our way back to our original life paths of enjoying our youth and making our own destinies. In my parent's old Lincoln, Patti and I would cruise Telegraph Road to pick up guys. Actually, Patti wouldn't quite put it that way. I'd roll her window next to some cuties in the next lane, throwing her into a panicked hello. She caught on fast, though, and loved these drag trips with the wind blowing through her short dark bob, flirting with men who would never know she was different. When boys would join us at the side of the road, we'd tell them we used wheelchairs and we'd chat up a storm. It was a thrill. We became involved in wheelchair sports, javelin, slalom, shot-put, and track. To this day I think I still hold a record or two. Patti became Miss Wheelchair Michigan 1974. Thick as thieves, we could be more magnanimous about the petty inconveniences of curbs and bathrooms, businesses and other people's parties. Our renewed independence outshone any major dispute we might have in our inaccessible communities.

On the other hand, Patti and I truly struggled with

any number of daily messages we received that we were an inconvenience to other people, or even worse, a convenience for them in telling lies about or distorting our lives as young women with disabilities. In Royal Oak one day, I remember one woman pointing us out to her preschooler as what she'd end up like if she didn't behave. It was so thoughtless, capturing the true stupidity of the time. In a strange way, this woman found it convenient to make use of us to emphasize the perils of poor behavior, as though Patti and I were little more than the riff-raff of society.

Once I set up an interview for an office position. My mom went with me because I wasn't sure how accessible the building would be. The supervisor came out and called my name, his gaze skipping over me toward my mother. When I said I was Cindy, a nervous look overcame him, replaced with a subtle scowl that I had not announced myself as disabled on the phone. I could definitely do this job, but his questions appeared obsessed with how inconvenient it would be for me to work there. How would I get to work? Could I be on time? Could I handle a desk job? Where was the ADA when you needed it? Needless to say, I didn't get the job. That man was mired in his inability to accept me for who I was and what I had to offer.

In a way, so was I. It took me a long time to accept that I would never walk again. Bull-headed, I tried to force my body how I wanted it to go. I borrowed Patti's splints and practiced walking along a set of parallel bars my father had constructed for me. I was able to pull myself up to a standing position, with my mother moving my feet along. When I showed the doctor and told him I wanted to walk with braces and crutches, his remark to me was "the only thing holding you up is willpower." I thought will was all I needed.

The problem with my will was that its exertion was overexerting my body. I couldn't just will things the way I wanted to. My body was not there as a matter of my own convenience as much as I wanted it to convey me places. I could not just act like it would be convenient to stand and walk one day and make that statement true. While this felt bad at the time, my attempts to walk also helped to define what I should expend my time and energy on. It was only then that I found it actually convenient to use my chair, since the comparison was no longer between rolling and walking but rather between getting there quickly and independently or being held as I struggled exhaustedly along.

To celebrate an inconvenient life you have to choose your battles and brag about every battle scar. There were battles I would fight to redefine convenient things as urgent life priorities. For example, driving represents not only the dignity of independent travel but also the means that most Americans connect functionally within adult society. Getting my chair in and out of the car was a challenge that with patience and determination became a mastered skill. I only managed to drop my chair and have it land on its side on the ground a few times over the years. Now that I was able to drive the world was my oyster even without its pearls of ease or thoughtfulness.

While it bothered me greatly, I accepted the limitations of freely visiting friends and family in their homes. It may seem superficial, even a luxury, to want to stroll over to your neighbors house for a quick cup of coffee or to have

Christmas at a favorite cousin's. In truth this inaccessibility is one of the primary causes of our growing isolation and frustration as people with SCI. The fact is that our communities are not universally designed. I can go to a dear friend's house to find that I can't transfer onto her toilet even though her house has ramps and she herself is a woman with a disability. I adjust myself to these inconveniences but cannot make peace with them. You see, I want in! I became very involved in barrier free legislation after learning firsthand what my future held.

Finally, there are times when inconvenience is just a convenient excuse to skirt other feelings and thoughts too uncomfortable for us to talk about, particularly but not limited to the details of our private lives. Personal inconveniences do play a very large role in my life and those of others with SCI or other disabilities.

The major two subjects of discomfort are bladder and bowel function, which will vary from person to person. I was extremely blessed with having both feeling and function in these areas. I was able to get rid of my catheter thirty six years ago. I like to think of the inconveniences that come from bowel and bladder as a kind of dark comedy, like unwanted houseguests who drop by your house and ruin your carpet. Things that I still have no control over when they decide it is time to visit are bladder infections and worse yet constipation or the dreaded "big D": diarrhea. You all know what I am talking about. It is hard enough for a walking person to make it to the bathroom. Try rounding corners on wheels to avoid the void.

Picture this: you are all ready to go out, shower taken, hair done, you're dressed in your favorite outfit, when all of a sudden you notice an aroma that doesn't smell like sweet soap or your favorite perfume. The literal exclamation of "oh shit" slips from your mouth as it coincidentally descends from your butt. The fact that you are not sitting on the toilet only accentuates the problem. Big inconvenience. People, this plane will be delayed for at least an hour. Really the inconvenient truth about our bodies after SCI is that we are like planes that sit on the runway. What mechanical problem will it be today? Pick up a good book and relax, for this is going to take time.

Your families may become familiar with these problems, but what about your able-bodied date who has never gone out before with a person with a disability? You are at the restaurant and have just ordered dinner. How do you explain to this stranger you really like that you have just pooped your pants? Dealing with embarrassment is the first challenge for most of us, followed by understanding or not, then acceptance or denial. We break with one of the grosser taboos every time our bodies do something completely good for them. You can only make certain choices about how you feel about your body, but you can behave in ways that present your bowels as an obstacle or as a temporary setback. What will you convey? What reality will you leave out?

Once you have passed this trial with loved ones, will others be as willing to volunteer to help? You will be surprised, but *yes.* I have been truly amazed at the number of times total strangers have asked if I needed help while I was in the restroom. This unbridled caring is a soothing salve for an otherwise upsetting situation. Cleaning up Baby is cute but the adult butt does not carry the same effect. Patti and I have waited for and helped each other in the public bathrooms for this very reason on many trips. Be assured that this may not the first or last time you will encounter the so-called inconvenience of public disability, but how you learn to deal with it will transform you from student to master.

My husband Tom will kill me for concluding with this tale, but it shows how having a sense of humor truly helps to exorcise the oppression we experience in our inconvenienced lives. One night, unbeknownst to me, my bowels decided to make a landing and not tell me. In the middle of the night, Tom rolled over and exclaimed (you guessed it) "oh, shit". Since he talks in his sleep all the time, I did not first pay too much attention. Then he moaned and raised the hand that had landed in the mess.

Now you have to understand that Tom's visceral tolerance for these things is actually on the low side. Slightly grossed out, he is always willing to help but has to get his wits about him first. I suppose that is why when he came out of the bathroom with a towel wrapped around his waist, one around his chest and one around his face, I totally lost it. I could have passed out from laughter. After that, I named him Dr. Pooh. The mess and lost sleep time were forgivable for us both, but Dr. Pooh was unforgettable. It was as though Tom had transformed himself in his honest way to address the sensitive and difficulty side of my injury, with love and for laughs. I felt glad to know him.

Then there are the bladder accidents that happen anywhere and everywhere. When you are sitting it is not quite so evident, hidden all under you. Eventually, however, whether you feel it or not, it will spread and start to smell. Preplanning is very important. You are on another date and you have a problem. Remember the plane? You hope your new friend is the patient kind because you are going to be delayed. I have missed several parts of movies and eaten cold food because of such inconvenience. Yet I am rarely the last person in the theater or the only one keeping people waiting. When I consider the particulars of my body now, there is a social meaning to its problems and uncertainties that so many other people share. I have come to realized that a very sizable portion of able-bodied society shares these same inconveniences also.

When you traverse this open-and-close world, it is important to get ahead of pesky inconveniences. History has taught me to be very specific. Break any obstacle you meet down into its inconvenience and consider the obvious and less obvious meanings attached to each inconvenience by you and others. Take inconvenience seriously: ask questions with purpose. Do you have a ramp and where is it located? Will I be able to enter from the front of the building? Is parking nearby? Are there any steps? How are the curb cuts? Are there automatic doors? Is there an attendant near the bathrooms? Is it very busy and noisy? May my friend or my personal care assistant come along? How long will we meet? Are you prepared to meet me, as the woman with a disability that I proudly am?

As I ponder over these last thirty eight years I have been truly blessed with excellent health, a fact for which I thank God every day. Patti is still a daily presence in my life, except now she is my sister-in-law. Over the last year I have been plagued with a buttock pressure sore that thinks it is my best friend, too. Friends like this I do not need. It hinders my ability to drive and come and go as I please because it opens up again and again as I transfer. This recent inconvenience has been personally challenging and soul searching for me because it is impinging on my precious independence. But get rid of my would-be best friend, this last unwelcome houseguest, and I will be good to go. There's no end to inconvenience in life, only the end of your rope or the end of one-way, have-it-all-now thinking. I have known both but find it more convenient to choose the latter.

4

DANNY HEUMANN

ON SEX AND MANHOOD

I want a better public vision of sex and disability. Before you get all bent out of shape, I am not a pornographer as much as a crusader. The vision I fantasize really starts with an adult sexual education film to show society that people with disabilities can enjoy amazing sex and fulfill their partners. We tend to think that people who have sustained a disability have lost the ability to have this quality of sex. Disabled men in particular can have great sex and the sex that women experience with us, given both the right chance and chemistry, probably is nine times out of ten better than sex that they have ever had before from able-bodied counterparts.

How can I make this boast? To the point, my disability makes a straight line between my body and my desires for another. It makes me think about what I need to do to please my partner. Disability and male sexuality are linked in the sense of achievement we get from satisfaction of all sorts. The possibilities are so much more for me now. I am open to so many different things now that I see how crucial the details are. No more narrow-mindedness. Listen to Playboy radio and you'll hear that able-bodied people all over the place are looking for more in their sex lives, that there's something missing. As disabled people we know what's missing. We're prepared for that extra mile. It's a matter of showing what we're made of.

Murderball, a recent documentary about the lives of United States Quad Rugby athletes and other disabled people, talks about sex and the sort of video about sexuality several guys were all shown in rehabilitation. I was shown that same video. Their reactions ranged from depression or incredulous laughter. I think about such movies often because so many of us with spinal cord injuries have no clue about how to be our-selves sexually, even less how to be men. When I got hurt in 1985 at 18 years old, when I was in the morning of my life, I certainly thought the worst thing that could happen to me as a man had to be my SCI. My sexual experiences I could count on one hand; then all of a sudden I'm paralyzed from the chest down with no movement and no sensation, in the words of my doctor, a complete ASIA-A. I dealt with all the immediate issues of learning my adult body after SCI at the same time like trying to remain a normal young adult who wanted a lot of sex with girls. Back then I wanted all those bodily experiences in college.

What was so sad was that college for this particular young disabled man became a massive fantasy. Figuring largely into this fantasy of manhood was playing sports passionately with my friends, something that before my injury I had loved to do. Specifically I loved basketball, to be on a court with nine other guys, running back and forth, talking trash. I sat there, part of it yet also not part of it. At Syracuse University, basketball was *the* male bonding experience. To sweat, to take all my anger and joy and let it flow out of my limbs as we ran, to experience that fast rejuvenation-- all this seemed suddenly gone from my body's possibilities. After classes, the guys would get together and play. That I couldn't do this felt so painful for me. What later felt like a miracle of self-discovery felt to me then like I was hitting the wall. Heck, I could see the wall as I was hitting it. To me it was all bullshit. I thought about suicide.

I was also really good at tennis, passionate about it, actually; it was cathartic. Like many men, I have loved my physical ability to send the ball in with an unquestionably good mark. Like sex, sport helps build my confidence and control, giving me a sense of my humanity. So after my SCI, I felt like a caged animal watching the rest of the pack go by, seeing others do things and not doing them myself. Yet it took fourteen years for me to pick up a tennis racket again, because emotionally I didn't want to play in a wheelchair. I felt it was accepting my disability, and I didn't want to accept it. Having to play in a wheelchair touched on my vulnerability as a man with a disability. I thought I never could play at the same level, the same veracity that I did before. I didn't like all the discussion about adaptive sports, for every time you wanted to do something that it had to be adapted. I didn't want to accept my disability, so why would I want to adapt to it?

The sport I finally got into after my disability, the one that really provided a sense of freedom for me, was sailing, because it was just me and the wind. I felt not only free but like a man. I sailed the Freedom-Independence, an adapted boat that was part of a second-phase rehabilitation program in Newport, Rhode Island. Sailing was our major recreational activity. It was great to get out there and compete against my fellow disabled sailors. On a Tuesday night, there would be eight of us out on different boats on the waves of the Naragansett Bay. Nature didn't care about our disability, and treated us like everybody else. For me that was freedom. Every time we went out on our sailboats, the most beautiful sight for us all was the tidy row of wheelchairs on the dock with nobody in them. *Empty chairs with nobody in them*: the dock was like that intermediate place in life between disability and freedom, and that was where we made our transformations.

We revitalized and told ourselves, even in light of our disabilities, that we were worthy of being productive in society. When I ultimately returned to land and my chair, I felt a "can-do" attitude that I could achieve anything I'd like in life. Think about this change for a moment: months before I had been lying in acute rehab at the Rusk Institute in Manhattan as an in-patient, my own private Riker's Island, thinking "what will my life be like now?" Who would think that a year and a half later Danny Heumann would be sailing the Naragansett Bay? Broken body afloat, captain of my own ship. The last thing I would ever dream was that I would be out on a beautiful sunny day on the same waters they sail for the America's Cup. In a million years at that point, I could never have thought of that.

When I think back that first attempt at free thinking about my body and my masculinity was really a gift from God, because that experience alone helped me believe that I could still have wonders in my life, like having my daughter now. I say "despite" now because disability to me is something associated with chains and shackles. For twenty years I have been tearing away at those chains and shackles. Real life with spinal cord injury includes lots of pit stops - lots of unexpected circumstances. With an SCI one moment you're doing an amazing activity and the next moment, because you've done this amazing activity, you've developed a stage-two pressure sore. My experience has been that every time you take two steps forward, something pulls you four steps back, an ebb and flow. It takes a real man (or a real woman) to leave the chair metaphorically behind and to navigate body and mind with a damaged nervous system.

Something about the chair still some days makes me feel like less of a man: I cannot do some things that an able-bodied man can do and I'm extremely jealous of that. Part of why I watch sex on video is to build up my own frustration while feeding my dreams voyeuristically, hoping and fantasizing that some day I will have it all again. Once I was there. Some of that immediately gratifying sexiness has been lost. Many days I still want my sensation back. It is part of my agenda in advocating and funding spinal cord research. Sharing this loss with you is not at all easy, but if we are not honest about our losses as men with spinal cord injuries, how can we be honest about the manhood we have, even less how we have gained sexually after SCI?

Sex *is* different for me. I would prefer to enjoy my impulses with the fluidity I might enjoy during intercourse. Sex requires production. We men don't like to think about that. But it is true. Now I think about how we arrange pillows and make plans at my house. The fact is that in my marriage, there are so many times I want take control over sex and not plan. Viagra can only take you so far, but don't tell that to Pfizer. It can't put you in the right place at the right time. It takes care of function but not emotion, not the pleasure, and not the positioning, and truly not the whole act, only one aspect of the act. The control is still not there.

So I have adapted my sexuality as a disabled male. I live in the real world. I could sit here every day cursing the world and say I can't do this or that. Instead I come to grips with what I can do. The reason I'm sitting in a wheelchair is not to be this aggressive man. I consider myself now a Pablo Picasso. Every time I would go to bed with a woman, I would paint a masterpiece. Now, of course, I'm lucky to working with one model. I love my wife. I explore the mental stuff and think a lot about the impulsive movement I want to do and thought I couldn't. It is challenging. The whole dynamic must change in terms of sensuality. Lack of intimate, unmediated sensation, like hot breath or that little playful nip, can be another painful wall unless we become more seasoned sexually as men, turning to the sensuality instead that our wives and partners crave.

For a woman married to a man with an SCI, as my wife has told me, fun, pleasing, and sensual sex is what she has found with me, something she had never had before. Attention to sensuous detail replaces mechanical sensation as only the means to an end. With SCI there is rarely the missionary position, then a quick goodnight. A quickie is usually not in the picture. And sometimes sex with SCI can be frustrating. Not much is easy with spinal cord injury. But when we give sex its due, it can be so fulfilling. If we want to be players and live our sex lives to the fullest, it is sexier to confront and own your situation. Accept your sex life. And make the most out of it.

Break out of whatever cage you are in, even the ones you have inherited from others. From my upbringing in a rigid New York Jewish household, I couldn't imagine my own father expanding his sexual repertoire. I had been conceived by my own parents in Israel in a sort of post-Holocaust parable of sexuality, a "miracle child" for two people who symbolically thought they would never be permitted to join in the beauty and celebration of heterosexual reproduction. I at least shared my father's respect for the sacredness of sex. In the last five years of his life my father became my best friend. Nonetheless, I have needed to expand my ideas of sexuality.

Many of us were at a disadvantage sexually even before our disabilities happened. A different generation handed me my morals and values about sex and about what manhood means. I was lucky to grow up not entirely in the dark, since I could pick up cues about myself from the savvy of New York City. When I was in rehab, before I had an actual post-SCI sexual experience, however, that savvy was turned on its head. I went from having all the answers to having none. The aides would tease me that now I'm a "cripple in a wheelchair", a nice Jewish boy who didn't know shit about shit about life, even less living with my injuries, even less about sex. Late at night while they would change my catheter and bathe me, they would tell me how my penis will never work, how I better learn (they would repeat this again and again) how to perform orally. That's what a man in a wheelchair does, my attendants would tell me, terrible news to a teenager who still thought that a woman's private parts were an undiscovered country.

The whole thought of it emasculated me. In the meantime, the sex films they showed us in the hospital were just horrible to look at. The women in the film were by movie standards ugly, the guys with SCI so shriveled and skinny it was depressing. We're talking too much hair and fungal toenails. Ben Vereen narrated how great sex was going to be, like Chicken George himself (I remembered him from *Roots*) is going to turn me on. Give me a break. Now that I've got an SCI, thought the teenage Danny, I'm like this guy in the film. Joe Quad having the old ear nibbled in the shower. I still remember every embarrassing detail. I consider it part of my trauma.

Twenty years later, I still think the movies they show to newly disabled people can be gross, bewildering, and depressing. These clinical videos hurt us even more than our SCIs, the affliction of our pain and suffering extended to our maleness. Should our sexuality be treated as a clinical experience? How can rehab help us to become the flesh-craving men that we are? Newly injured, I was looking for what was true about life. We need support in exploring the distinction of having sex following disability. If I had seen a good raw sex film, I would have felt differently about my future as a man with an SCI.

When Christopher Reeve talked to the scientists, he did not talk about sex or how difficult his bowel movements were on a given day, but *we* need to do this. Since our privacy becomes a public subject for them, we must push for a full range of options. We can make decisions about how we have sex, just like scientists do with their own partners, so when these scientists go back to their Petrie dishes they remember what we deserve: a cure or a treatment so we can enjoy the Full Monty.

Reaching deep into our sexual identities as men with SCI, we also encounter sexualities that appear trivial but are not. We grow up with this whole Madison Avenue concept that sex equals beauty. I know its limits, but I appreciate its honesty. What's most ugly about my disability is my lack of control over my abdomen, because it just sits there like a lug. I don't like saying I love something that, regardless of my conditioning, I dislike. But my eyes are still open and wanting, and my life is still happening. I want to think both outside and inside the Madison beauty box. I want what I want. To achieve this, I actually need to contradict the low expectations by society given to our male sex lives and the importance of fantasy to us. So I want to see good-looking women in chairs and put them into our popular culture, with good-looking guys in chairs, complete with that fabulous anything-goes Madison Avenue concept. The sky is the limit.

Now America loves reality TV, but when a boy with SCI is eighteen years old, he honestly does not want that reality that much. Non-disabled young men can take or leave concepts of sexuality until they are more mature. Since we are confronted with being disabled, we still need our fantasies to get us through. Even if they are not realistic in life, sexual fantasies help adapt us to our injuries. We see that a hot sex life is still possible and that there are men and women in chairs living that life.

The way we talk about disability and sexuality, however, is still full of negativity and despair. Why do we think in the disability community there's overuse of drugs, alcohol, tobacco? Because under those influences perhaps we numb ourselves. We get stoned before sex to relieve our inhibitions around spinal cord injury and sex. Or we dwell on sad truths, like Tom Cruise in *Born on the Fourth of July* when he's in a Mexican brothel with a prostitute. He's crying because he can't feel her. That scene in that movie says it all.

But if we want to live life, we have to get away from that despair. How sad it was that he couldn't feel himself inside of her, so symbolically painful that this was his new life and reality. To this day, I can see that scene and still cry. Like with that rehab film, we're told all we can do is lay down. That's not even true. There's more. When two people are pulled up together and hold onto each other, they still feel themselves as one. Sex can still be really good.

If you choose to stay home and curse the world, nobody will care. The sun will rise and set and you will be the loser. You'll miss out on relationships and great sex. So will the loves of your life. For the first ten years of my injury I let my disability control me, and I lived in denial of both. Once I figured out that my wheelchair would get me from Point A to B in all things, including my sexual happiness, I stopped letting my paralysis define me. Danny had to become Danny again. And that is why I have been able to build a marriage and have a child.

This is how my disability has challenged my virility. As the Grateful Dead write in "The Wheel": "Small wheel turning by the firing rod/ Big wheel turning by the grace of God/ Every time the wheel turns around/ I'm bound to cover just a little more ground." Sex for us men is naturally about desire, about getting more, feeling better, learning more, challenging ourselves. Pushing ourselves to the limit and over. Game on.

5

THOMAS HOATLIN ON FAITH

I don't think a lot of people in the world slow down to contemplate the goodness of themselves. When I speak in public, I talk about what happened to me and all I have been through, then say, "Isn't that remarkable!" Then I ask, what is your remarkable? At least could you stand up here like me and say are your blessings? Obviously it wouldn't be, as happened to me, getting shot in an armed robbery and being left with paraplegia. At first this wouldn't be a blessing for anybody. But your blessing might be successfully raising four children. It might be dealing with a difficult teenager or your own substance abuse. It might be getting through divorce and coming out brighter on the other side. It might be coping with the loss of a partner or a parent. Somehow, despite personal tragedies and catastrophes, some of us manage to keep living with an eye always on what is remarkable. So what is your remarkable? If you don't have one, could you search one out? Could you create one? Could you start working on it?

To find the remarkable takes a lot of faith. We all need to learn how to see our lives as remarkable. By remarking on what graces our lives after spinal cord injury, we enjoy the very most of why we are here on Earth. I ask people to concentrate and recollect times in their lives when goodness triumphs over sadness because to remember the goodness is to prevail over suffering. Goodness may come in an instant or will work its way into our lives over time. My work at the Ann Arbor Center for Independent Living has given me the opportunity to inquire about people diverse in characteristics both in the community and at the hospital. I have discussed remarkable things with residents, parents, people with new spinal cord injuries, students, and friends with SCI. The actual premise or ideology remains the same: what is remarkable connects in us what is worthy in ourselves with what *today* we are able to do. We tend not to be aware of what forces transform abstract goodness into the concrete well-being of our personal lives. Simply, it is hard to evaluate and realize good things for ourselves. We neglect ourselves. We don't mark the tiny positive changes that are within our grasp, good things that we can actually see and feel in the real world. But when we do make this connection between a world we function in today and the potential in us to do something worthwhile in that day in this world, that's remarkable.

Finding what is remarkable in your life defines your faith. In the context of traumatic spinal cord injury, however, a devastating transformation often comes suddenly and violently. It is hard to mark your adjustment since so much happens so fast. What are our new baselines? What will be our new benchmarks? If we can't mark our beginnings, it is nearly impossible to map what is remarkable for us. We don't know where to go. Some of us forget even how to feel good. Though I am generally a positive thinker, it was so easy to forget. I can map the exact date and nature of my permanent injury as well as the fact that I cannot move my hips or legs. Like trying to start a dead battery on a car, except my situation was not remediable with a new battery or a new spinal cord, my life at first appeared "remarkable" only for having been broken.

Some of us end up in the dumper if our lives get reduced to these "remarkable" but negative characteristics, however powerful they may seem. Just because we have been terribly injured does not mean we should give in to destructive forces. It is up to us to interpret the change in our lives following spinal cord injury, to interpret the traumas and to decide whether they can be transformed into something remarkable for *good*.

When someone with a spinal cord injury gets worked up over an access problem that separates him or her from a previous way of living, something that leads to a pure sadness, I share my own parallel experience. I remark to them how, just years before, my new losses appeared insurmountable, for example, how frustrated I would get when faced with physical barriers. Not being able to access every inch of the earth is part of my life now, it is part of every day, and I choose not to fight every accessibility battle. Instead I look at the access I do have and remark to myself that today, this may be good enough. Not being able to do things I used to or and have what I have lost can turn explosive in mind, body, and soul. I have learned to pick my battles.

Unfortunately, many people are quite negative, whether they have spinal cord injuries or not. They don't even realize they are being negative. They are clearly not able to see many blessings or the small things that might make them feel at peace. The power of letting it go is amazing, that leap of faith everyone talks about but rarely makes. The power of saying something nice about someone you had ignored can also be both liberating and enriching. The power of taking back your life, well, gives you back your life.

For me, this was more than a lesson in self-evaluation. Case in point: one gunshot during an armed robbery at a suburban hotel in 1991 left me paralyzed from the chest down, needing a wheelchair for mobility, and experiencing a new vulnerability. Two years of marriage, a new baby girl, a first family Christmas in our starter home—basically a life rich with blessings—were all catastrophically interrupted. Two men, my worldly opposites, intentionally did evil things, including leaving me to die. What happened to me is what most people only experience in a nightmare. Later a policeman reported that I saved my own life, crawling beneath the customer service counter rather than lying open on the office floor as I was told to do by my assailants.

Still, one moment and my life was different. Was that remarkable in itself—that I lived? In that moment there was extreme pain. My hand came away from my neck with a great gush of maroon blood. In the next hour I lost twelve units, nearly all I had in my body. In the hours that followed, my freedom to go anywhere, do anything for a while also was drained away. Instead of Christmas, instead of serenity, I spent half a year in the hospital, fearful and fighting for my life.

For the first couple of months, I had such an attitude. I lost faith in the things I had right in front of me. In the hospital on Christmas Eve, the doctors came in with their "wonderful" gift of telling me that I would never walk again. As they left, carolers came down the hallway. I asked a visitor to slam my door shut really loudly. The weekend before the robbery I had just decorated the lobby of the hotel with poinsettias, garland roping with red ribbon, and a huge, evergreen wreath over the grand fireplace mantel. Christmas had been my favorite time of year, a time of giving and sharing, being off work and being with family. I found it hard during that December to believe that I could ever feel that holiday comfort and excitement ever again. I engaged in the negativity of my own thoughts during that time, and when I did, a lot of it was hatred toward my perpetrators, the men who had robbed me of mobility and spirit. While they went to prison for thirty-five years, I felt I was in the prison of my chair for life.

Over time I came to realize that none of us are prisoners of our chairs. None of us are "wheelchair bound". We are just not. My life isn't my disability. My life is about living. People have told me that they forget I even have a disability. While I am proud to be disabled, I forget this, too. We are people who use wheelchairs the way we use other things. Our chairs are simply our bodies' vehicles, what keeps us out in the community, replacing for some of us who have paraplegia, two legs with four wheels, and for others with quadriplegia, legs and arms with wheels and supports.

Just this shift in thinking alone didn't dissolve my negativity, however. This started with other good things, to be more precise, doing good things and feeling well in them. Time with my baby daughter, keeping up with her fast-paced needs, occupied me so much that at the end of the day I could say in sheer exhaustion that I am her father. I wanted to be a role model. My mother told me I had two choices: work toward my recovery in physical therapy, or stay miserable and make everyone around me miserable. She didn't believe for a moment that I would choose the second. I hear that from patients in the hospital now. They tell me they are going to be okay because they just don't have a choice. We can't go back and undo our spinal cord injuries.

I have seen people, five and ten years after injury, choose misery. Their misery dehumanizes them, steals their spirits, puts their bodies' gas tanks on empty, and crushes their dreams and goals. Certainly my blood boils when barriers present themselves, with hotels that know I'm coming and argue with me over what makes a room "accessible". But that's different: it's all right to feel anger over what has happened to us and what barriers continue to block our ways as we wheel through the world. It is up to us to make this world accessible, to do whatever it takes. But for others who allow their spirits to remain stolen, this can lead to very dark places. This is when faith can become a guiding light in the dark. This is when a seemingly unremarkable person can become remarkable.

It took some time for me to realize that my faith, as I had known it, had been lost with the attack on my body. Where there's faith, there is hope, always, unwavering, and unconditional. So while faith was taken from me, it is the one thing I could recover one hundred percent. Having faith in God sustains me and helps me to realize my self-worth and my goodness.

We are all here as a vocation. We are servants, if you

will. To act on our vocations can be so fulfilling, so nurturing, feeding into the quality of our lives in literal and spiritual ways. That makes us remarkable. We are all needed. You may not have met your vocation, but it will come, if you seek it.

Extending our faith after spinal cord injury does not need to be done formally or traditionally. It can be felt and thought and taken and given any number of ways, day or night. I can look to a friend who also has SCI and take it on faith that my difficult experience can be understood, even empathized with. I can offer a little prayer, and all of a sudden the tension of my day seems broken up. If anything, my SCI has taught me that one does not just have faith, just like one doesn't just exist. But we must train ourselves to look for the goodness and to believe in it. Faith itself is remarkable. Faithful acts feed into the quality of our lives in literal and spiritual ways.

Why not take ten whole minutes of every day and pray silently or out loud? Pray to whomever you wish, God, someone who's gone before you, or yourself. Do something. We are here for a very short, short time. Children don't always grow up. Men and women don't always reach their seventies. Blessings seem to evaporate sometimes. I should and could be only an angry person for having lost a baby and two friends before I was thirty, and then year after year of tragedy, getting shot by two strangers. For my faith, I am more remarkable.

Truthfully, I lost a big chunk of my faith for a while. It's been a journey back, one that has been very worth the trip. My faith is back but with more richness. Without faith, I would not be whole today. I would not say that my life with spinal cord injury is always happy or always good, for that matter. But my life with SCI is nearly always faithful. I needed to become this person of deeper faith, someone who can be called upon to extend my hand to others who know the terrible depths of living unremarkably with SCI. Because without faith, no matter how steady or turbulent our faith is, we lose the hope for our survival and the chance for our greatness.

6

Although it has defined my life, risk to me is difficult to put into words. As a young person, I was the typical kid who felt indestructible. I grew up climbing trees fast and competing for the highest leap. On skates or go-go cart, I would grab the back fenders of moving cars, a daredevil to myself and others. My lack of concern continued as a teen-ager and young man, never having had broken bones or operations. Years went with no thoughts on my part of becoming injured. I never had to go to the doctor except for my pre-season athletic exams. I had a false sense of security, since I seemed able to do all these things without being hurt, even though friends would break their arms or twist their ankles. I felt different from them and let my luck go to my head. I felt blessed.

My dad was an exceptional athlete, and I had been given the same sorts of abilities. Smaller than other children my age, six or seven inches shorter, I could beat them at running the football down the field, blocking for teammates without hesitation. I thought I was mighty special. I told myself not to get too egotistical but let my actions do that for me. I elevated myself even more, saying that my accomplishments were normal for me. I had grown accustomed to coming out in first place. Losing was not part of my vocabulary.

As I grew older, I thought I grew out of doing these childish and dangerous things. I began weighing my risks in middle or high school. I knew my friends were insane to experiment with modified BB or Zip guns. I knew accidents would happen with twenty two bullets. I also knew I was too small to go out for varsity football so opted for cross country instead. After a year of it, though, I saw that running was good conditioning for wrestling, a sport where I would not be riding the bench. Immediately satisfying to me, no one was able to pin me to the ground. Wrestling was an individual challenge, just me against an opponent in front of an audience. As a junior and senior I felt like a gladiator with everyone applauding me as I cradled or guillotined some poor guy, putting him in a banana split, fireman's carry, or half Nelson.

The truth of that glorious time when I walked the halls with pats on the back and girls doing their little flirty thing, was that I grew distracted from the reasoning I needed to make good decisions. Some risks never stand out as much as others; and our human desire tends to obscure those risks even more. Commonly wrestlers would pick a weight fifteen or twenty pounds less than normal in order to wrestle their best. We wanted to be muscle and bone. Some of the ways of cutting weight to make one's class were quite risky. In fact, some are illegal now. I would put on the rubber suit and layers of clothing before practice or "dry out" by eating a couple of ice cubes for dinner with a Lifesaver for dessert. Every once in a while in the newspaper we'd read that some local wrestler had died from exactly such overexposure, weight loss, dehydration, or malnutrition. Not going to happen to me. I felt nothing, never felt near death. I ignored every sign of danger. My fingers would cramp into fists from lack of sodium. In the minutes before matches, I needed alcohol rubbed on my clubbed hands to relax them. My hands did not feel dangerous, although the reason for their tightness was. But I wanted to succeed so much that I would change any way I could for the win.

Risk is such a natural part of childhood. The older you get, the wiser, the more knowledgeable of risk you become, but for the young adult in all of us, risk is not something you can reach out and really look at. It is invisible to our psyches because we are submerged in our passions and in our childlike needs to win. We can look back and see how dangerous our childhoods were. We grow more conscious of this and tell our kids to watch out and be careful. Except for my dad, no one told me to watch out. I would tell kids at school not to jump from buildings, not to climb to the highest branches to get the kite that's already ripped to shreds, not to climb out on life's limb without caution. We hold on with one hand to a twig not much bigger than our fingers, the other hand reaching out for the kite, just because we can do it. We do it often, and we are lucky to be alive.

Ironically, my first spinal cord injury came from the very thing I felt secure in. At the time I was injured, I was performing a particular wrestling hold, resisting at fifty percent strength, working on the particular move. My practice opponent gave back too much resistance, more than what he should. I fell. And he fell on my head. If one does it right, this accident rarely happens. I trusted him to do a particular hold, but in the spirit of team initiation, this man meant to haze me in surprise. I like to think of it as an initiation because it represented to me a rite of passage, earning my place among my teammates. This was a rite that went wrong. I dislocated my neck. I couldn't move or breathe. I was scared to death. In eighteen years, it was my first serious injury of any sort, a mess of hospitalization and rehabilitation.

Suddenly risk shifted in meaning, and that bothered

me. Though I felt stunned and hurt at being told I could never wrestle again, that walking was at 200 to 1 odds, as time went on my body healed and forgot. I did start walking. Nurses fed me while that invincibility crept back in. This, too, would pass. I would be all right. It would be just a matter of time. I was ignorant of my injury's long term impact. I looked at this accident as a negative mark on my reputation.

I was the exception to the odds and the learning. My machismo led me to think I would bounce right back and carry on as I always had. Others like me were only interested in being the best, not in being realistic, not in overdoing things. There weren't any signs that I had overdone anything. The only sign I got from the surgery was that my spinal cord had been smaller than normal, and now it was stronger because of the cervical fusion. Why not take more chances? My life, like that of almost any young and gifted adult, meant competition; the desire to win overwhelmed my thinking. But as soon as you put your hand on the hot stove, you would think you would learn not to do it again. Mine was a freak accident, though, not to be repeated. I was not numbskull enough to keep wrestling with the team, yet I did not become more careful or thoughtful.

I was more upset that I couldn't wrestle than that I was learning how to walk. I had no idea what winning could mean. I only wanted it. In my dorm room I would spar with my roommate, who was the state's wrestling champion in his higher weight class. (I was champion in mine.) We were grapplers, the kind of kids that, regardless of where we were, we would have to get into it. I thought about my doctor's advice to quit or stop, but would only do so when I had the advantage over the guy. If I were under him, I never thought of my neck or spine. Controlling my life through risk taking took over the lack of control I might have felt as a man who had broken his neck.

In comparison, my next twenty-seven years appeared to be smooth sailing. I built a family and completed my education at the same time. My lifestyle changed with having a son and a daughter who needed me. For most of their lives I was a single parent without child support. I did fewer risky things, pointing out to my children the same hazards my father had shown me. I thought I had come of age, that I understood risk in the limited sense that certain actions were to be avoided.

Risk, however, is everywhere and in everything, an unfastened seatbelt, playing catch with a child, eating too fast. Even with some wisdom, I still played rough-tough with my kids and drove home from the bar high from Jack Daniels. Part of me changed with increasing maturity and experience, and part of me stayed in denial of my mortality. I could not know all the details that make me now a survivor, an excellent former athlete, a strong man, a father who has seen both his children go to college.

Risk is like light and shade. We become enlightened from being faced with memories of who we were and how we would like our children to survive this potentially disastrous world. Anyone can be swallowed up in this world, from dangers—partying, fighting, bullets, crack, drive-by's, knives in school, killing—that were not part of my youth but are part of our children's lives as I write this now. Yet we are also shaded from understanding risk. Risk can bankrupt you, cost you friends, wreck marriages. In short, risk can be positive or negative, the gamble of going up to the right young lady, the possibility of being denied, the embarrassment at being told no, but the chance of ending up getting married. Risk is spending your last ten dollars on a lottery ticket. As time went by, after divorce and in an empty nest, more and more I bought lottery tickets and, often, alcohol. That's when I hit rock bottom. Since alcohol loves company, an alcoholic friend would break from his factory job at three o'clock in the afternoon, and we would get bottles of beer from the local store. He would get crazy drunk, and I would join him.

There are large and small ways risks are good for us, making us more durable in our plans to live full and responsible lives. But is it okay to look for the good in bad risk? Even my riskiest act, the one I know only because the words "spinal cord injury" tell me was really, really bad—even this act could have been worse. Drunk driving was a bad decision, and I feel badly about it, but part of me based my risk on another calculation that I would rather drive my daughter's car than risk her safety. Truth is, the car was working but not my ability to drive it. This was not just an accident. I thought I was buckling my seatbelt with both hands, steering with my knees, but because of the car's wrecked suspension, I was fumbling with my life as the car veered left.

Now I'm at the other side of that decision. And I have come back to wrestling, this time wrestling with the meaning of my accident and the reality of my addiction. During the year after my second spinal cord injury, I woke up and got my wits together. It was like *deja vu*, but this time I knew I'd done some irreparable damage to my body. My parents were much older than they were when I had had my first injury, so I wondered if they could take it again.

My father had been so hurt by my original SCI, worried for his son to be completely paralyzed, dependent on others, no longer an athlete. After my second SCI, he was devastated, both my parents were. No one had to tell me. I just knew. I was in really bad shape. Because I was no longer youthful or powerful, my father had to grieve the loss of my abilities in 1991, twenty seven years after my first accident in

1964. Remember he was an athlete of Olympic caliber, having set the world record in the 400 meter hurdles once upon a time. My father's love for me had translated into our shared athleticism. He had seen me following in his footsteps, excelling at golf, winning championships, breaking records. In this I could not follow any more.

My second SCI also meant a great, disruptive shift both in responsibilities and common sense in relation to my parents and children. I wrestled with the last years of my parents' lives, feeling horrible about what they may have been feeling about my disability, despite their protests that they were happy I was alive. Even as my father deteriorated into dementia, he would visit me at home on special occasions, and he seemed more secure for the good marriage I had made with Karla.

I felt relieved to see them move on in their lives as I began to move on in mine. I didn't miss a beat, returning to my career as a school counselor. In his last days, my father seemed happy for me again, and I took pleasure in showing him that I still had a good mind and was functional. I like to think that he left feeling that I was normal, able to do what other normal people can do. But in the back of my mind I felt terrible that I had done such stupid things, so much risk-taking that I really hurt and disappointed them. I felt embarrassed.

I learned that I have opponents that weigh far more than I do. Risk of rushing, risk of safety, risk of addiction: could I still put them to the mat? Now I take a tenth of the stupid risks that I used to, recovering from my alcoholic ways and childish daring. I no longer think I know better than the laws of the physical universe. I finally learned that such risk can kill you. I knew my body could not tolerate alcoholic intoxication any longer, so nipped a full-blown addiction in its flower. My second SCI made me really size up and come to grips with all sorts of risks. To be the right kind of role model for my grown children and my students, I knew I had to remove the tarnish of my earlier, lackluster ways. The pinnacle of my embarrassment came with the memory that I had for many years taught driver's education, and I imagined my former students in their grown up lives talking to their friends about their driving teacher driving with both hands off the wheel.

I began counseling kids about the risks they take, explaining the laws of nature. For my at-risk youths to even be here, I would tell them, they were fortunate enough to have already survived a risky life. I would explain to them that there were many people who were no longer here because of such risks, driving ninety miles an hour in the snow, drinking or drugging themselves to the point of false security, believing themselves indestructible. How could they foresee the consequences of such risks? The young and the daring will think that they can do anything they want in any way that they imagine.

I knew my one match was over, with both shoulders pinned to the floor, when my teenagers would hear about what happened to me. We usually didn't need much spoken language; eye contact in the hallways was often enough. I know about you, or, you're important to me, their eyes would say. The wrestlers in particular knew I had been a star, and they knew I hadn't returned for the salary. I wouldn't teach or preach but rather help them form new ideas and make their own decisions, that no matter how tough they were that they may falter over the issue of risk. In a different sort of rough-toughing, with some guys, I would refer to Superman, someone who in real life had acquired a disability from falling from his high perch-- someone whose invincibility was a myth. I hope they believe me. Kids tell my wife if not for her husband they would not have made it. Karla and I believe them, and our arms open wide. This is the spark that keeps me alive. The more I see these young African-American men, the less I feel paralyzed.

Nowadays I feel prouder. I have lived one heck of life and plan to live as long as I can. I would like to continue to be myself. I have no interest in acting wild and crazy. I don't need to be Superman. I am beyond the myth; I have stopped trying to be someone past my own reach, beyond my normal abilities to succeed. I am a role model instead of a drunkard. I am here for a purpose. Few people break their neck twice without getting their wits together.

Some individuals never really outgrow risk, constantly

looking for something, continuing to drink or speed, anything they can repeat over and over again. They tire of what they can tolerate, looking for ways to get out. They do it because they still can and will continue to do this, even as their friends perish at the same risk.

Starting a new business, looking at something new, something I may not excel in—in short, finding a true challenge—that defines risk for me now. I am thinking of going down to Alabama to see my nine-year-old grandson, risking my wheelchair on the airplane, for last time I flew, when I went to the Bahamas, they let my chair fall, breaking my power box. But if I don't go, I may suffer from something even more dangerous, the consequences of staying home too much and away from the ones I love. When my daughter's husband was killed in a motorcycle accident, I missed being there for her and my grandchild. Time goes by quickly, and as risk-takers love to say, there are no guarantees. Togetherness, being part of activities, can become depleted as we isolate ourselves, limiting our sense of where we can and cannot go. I have learned to pay more attention to every possibility that

DEEP

could bring me closer to my loved ones.

I could still be sitting around feeling sorry for myself. This sort of risk is a matter of losing control over my destiny. Once upon a time, I responded to my son and daughter's distress calls. Now I need my family here for me, and if I do not ask for this sort of closeness, I risk our happiness. I also risk my ability to continue asserting my identity as a man, a husband, a father, a role model, an educator, and an elder. I am still searching for the respect for all that I am. And I need to admit that I now need their nurturing. Does this mean I am less strong? No. As I recognize their respect in my life as it is today—in my son's memories of our runs around the block or my daughter's "Thank you, Daddy." I can turn their nurturing comments and actions into the strength I need to live today with dignity.

I don't want to hear someone else saying, "Poor soul" or "That Charles. He'll never be the same again." I am still an individual with feelings so get upset with how much I have to surmount to access my home or neighborhood safely. Charles should have learned his lesson. Now my objective is to get ahead of the risk, rather than operating without a brain or a net.

Two summers ago, at my fortieth class reunion, folks gathered around as though I were a completely different person. As they expressed their sympathies, I could feel I was no longer their great hope, their star athlete. My voice wasn't even strong enough for them to hear the answers to their echoes of "How did this happen to you?" I am not sure I understood my answers to their questions. How could I be both this man in a wheelchair and come from the proud stock of African-American men in my community? When I was inducted into the Ypsilanti High School Athletic Hall of Fame in 2005, prior inductees milled around me, uncomfortably shaking their heads. They had looked up to me. Now I could see their pitying thoughts. How can people respect me when they pity me? That's the paradox.

These reactions keep me somewhat withdrawn. I grow shyer and shyer. The tension between who I was and who I am physically still bothers me: half of me enjoyed the adulation of the public while another half of me loved the privacy in caring for my lawn and garden, watching things grow under my strong, gentle, broad fingers. Mine was a vise grip. Neither half of my former physical self is there now. I do not visit friends in their homes. I do not cut my own grass, weed, or plant flowers. As tedious as those tasks might seem, I miss them. I could continue with this contradiction endlessly, for while I love having my life, I also have lost the life I could most appreciate in myself. I know I do not need my legs in order to be worthy. But I do need to do some more work still. My biggest hold-back is my mental attitude toward my hands and arms. I tend to define my hands by what I can no longer do, greet someone at the door, embrace my wife, scribble notes for my paperwork.

It feels both great and terrible to keep scores at the tournament named for me, the Ypsilanti High School Beatty-Lambros Wrestling Invitational. It's difficult to say this, but sometimes I feel embarrassed to be in this chair, not just

because of the risks of too much alcohol and unfastened seatbelt, but because like them, I once represented a paragon of
African-American manhood. I see the boys wrestle and can
only guess what is not on their minds. Worse, I play these
games still with myself, this wrestling between self-pity and
self-respect that comes with my present state of being a fine
African-American man with a spinal cord injury. I used to
pity the good-looking men who hurt themselves, like their
lives after risk were complete wastes. No respect for the lives
we had, no respect for the lives we live know. There is life
after wrestling. After you pin your adversary to the mat, win
or lose, you must get up and walk to your next match.

    This afternoon I looked at my own hands and asked
myself if I had more self-respect or more self-pity for them. It
is a rough question to ponder. I feel bad about them, but I do
not pity them. I put them into the shape that they are, but if I
did not care about them, I wouldn't keep them in structuring
braces or do my range of motion exercises. My hands should
not be neglected; like the rest of me, they deserve my respect,
because they have survived every risk with me. Pity means to

me that I will never use these hands, when who knows what is around the corner. Athlete that I am, I am still training for the next event. I still make my wife nervous when I dash off over rickety bridges at the nearby park. I am just not ready to go yet in any sense of the word. I care for myself. My body is still a temple.

7

MARCY EPSTEIN ON HUMILITY

I should have been a pair of ragged claws
Scuttling across the floors of silent seas.

    T.S. Eliot, "The Love Song of J. Alfred Prufrock"

For in that sleep of death what dreams may come
When we have shuffled off this mortal coil,
Must give us pause.

    William Shakespeare, Hamlet

Relatively speaking, I have a very mild spinal cord injury, what is medically termed an incomplete SCI (ISCI) at C4-C5, functionally an "ASIA D." I breathe and eat on my own and on many days can walk with little pain. Compared with some of my friends with incomplete quadriplegia, I have few bladder problems and have not used a chair since the first month of my injury. My upper body is weaker than before and my nerves are jangled in ways made known only by pain, spasm, or tingling. My arms burn up daily, but I have come nearly to ignore it. I have been traumatized and twisted but see this as par for the course. In fact, except for those who stare at the jagged band of scar on my neck, most people are surprised to learn I have a disability. It is hidden like this story has been till now.

Many people might think my being in a no-man's land of SCI as a relief, this passing among the non-disabled, free from their pity or disparagement. Sometimes I feel like no other man. I know I don't have people staring at my wheelchair or my vent pack. It is painful when I am expected to hide my disability for a job interview because I *can*, because employers are statistically less likely to hire me if they believe I will make them install ramps and elevators in their old buildings. It upsets me to be questioned if I am disabled enough to warrant flexibility or compassion. I feel humiliated when I drop the bag I'm carrying in the middle of the store, get stuck in a sitting position, have someone else clean my sink, or miss a meeting. My ISCI makes me weary and different, abject and special in turns. I have an un-popular version of this disability, and I experience it as entirely curious, often difficult, and sometimes humiliat-ing.

Feeling humiliated is not an entirely horrible or isolated event for me. It is good to get over ourselves. For every thing I've lost that I've loved, there's another thing I'm glad to be rid of. Plus there are probably a few folks out there who think I have needed to come down a peg or two. I appear as a strong-willed and privileged person, a thin veneer that covers my sensitive, nearly doggish pack mentality. I think in the plural. *Myself is more than myself.* One could say I both lack and embody humility. Perhaps humiliation and humble-ness both relate to humility, the former in suffering and the latter in serenity. My ISCI has inspired humility in me. I ac-tually looked this word up in Merriam-Webster's dictionary to make certain I had the right word to describe my experience. *Humility*, it turns out, has two meanings, both of which describe the edgy sharpness that my spinal cord injury has added to the paradox of being humbled: first, humility implies "being brought down to a lower level" (now there's a literal description of what's happened to us!) and "forcibly make humble."

I struggle both with forces that humble me as well as with the humility itself. Paradoxically, I suffer with too much pride. The days before my injury offer a perfect example: with four hundred dollars of traveler's checks in my backpack to last four months, one week after graduating from a doctoral program at the University of Michigan, I set off through the Negev Desert and southernmost Israel, up through Jordan to Petra, and westward to the Old City of Jerusalem. At first, traveling through the Middle East to land at a *beit midrash* (house of interpretative study) for women seemed like a glorious immersion in a modest plan. I thought it was the education I really needed. I thought I was humbling myself. By the third bout of heat exhaustion and twentieth repetition of pita and hummus (pocketbread with chick-pea spread), I was dried out in all respects. Not much dignity is accorded a scrubby white American in khaki shorts sipping an iced tea for hours in an air-conditioned hotel bar. Even my modesty seemed unbelievable.

Most of my story of spinal cord injury has become peppered with an uncomfortable sense of humor about my attempts to get down and rugged after years in the Ivory Big House, as well as my inanity about my own importance in this tale. While it happened to me, my broken facets are also facets of other lives. Whose body lives and dies in seclusion? The day before I was injured I joined my brother Donald and our large family for his eldest son Charles's bar mitzvah at the Western Wall. I left the King David Hotel with its exquisite furniture for a single-sex hostel bunk among the *Lubavitchim*, a religious sect dedicated to a zesty renewal of religious practice among worldly youth. I was thirty-two. And crucially, at 10:30 the next morning, a Wednesday, I agreed against my better judgment to ride a camel up a cliff to a little desert dwelling called *Eretz Bereshit*, Land of the Beginning.

Had this been the camel's story, it might be short: "I threw some woman off of me and onto her head." My mother reminds me that the beast spat in my face afterward. Sadly, seriously, I have to own this story, since it is my spine that snapped, my body that felt myriad nerves pulsing and energy flowing in rivulets down into the sands. My mind came to as cousins and brothers ran over to shield me from the burning sun and Bedouin teenagers tried to stand me up. My voice said "*Lo—La'a—No*" in any language I could recall, any utterance to leave me be and so save my life. Land of the Ending.

Back to the dictionary for a breath of fresh air. Humility's second definition pokes right at my physical and philosophical spine and those two hours in the desert waiting for the ambulance to arrive. It means *to mortify*. I felt embarrassed to have fallen and strangely more embarrassed not to be able to get up and walk up to that tourist-trap lean-to and the rest of my life. I felt mortified to have ridden that camel at all, even more to need special attention from my family during its celebration of our first-born. Most important, I had *been* mortified.

Transferred quickly from one hospital to the regional center for neurological and orthopedic emergencies, like many of you, I nearly died. If I excise the layers of anxiety and trauma I also feel around such mortification, the experience of spinal cord injury is still a threshold journey between life and death. Some of us have even been revived from death. Just experiencing some of the conditions of death—swelling till we can no longer breathe, ceased sensation in our trunks and limbs, stilled agency or movement, the fluids seeping out of us—these experiences give us insight into life. We are molded, borrowing from Hamlet's to-be-or-not-to-be soliloquy, into "these mortal coils". Shakespeare wrote "mortal coils" to represent our whole bodies, which I like, but I also appreciate the specifics of the phrase. Our cords are those mortal coils. We are so tender and so complex that we might unravel, not to regain our shapes; we are also so tough and so tight that it takes a car crash, a high dive, an ornery camel, something universally powerful to uncoil us. Vented, cathed, paralyzed or petrified, we're not shuffled off yet.

Careful: I am not linking disability with death but rather disability with life. We have held onto life with tighter grips than working hands could ever muster.

It was sometime between Day 2 and Day 4 in the ICU, in a lull between shifts I would guess, that I lay in my own filth for about three hours. My voice box had swelled too much for me to be heard, so I cried from sheer exertion, stress, and embarassment. A woman, a hospital volunteer with her hair tied modestly back under her *snood*, heard my tears as she walked from bed to bed distributing fresh blankets. The bones of her fingers felt so cool and fragile as she lay her hand over mine, asking me what was the matter. "I've soiled myself," I rasped to her, grasping her hand softly, choking on tears and phlegm, "Please help me." My self-importance ebbed from me like a red tide, "I shouldn't be like this. I'm filthy. I can't reach. You have got to help me."

It occurred to me then that she did not have to help me. Who was I to her? No one in her job description. The Israeli health system is not consumer-centered, either; I barely figured into their picture of a typical day of traffic mortalities and bomb victims, emergency technicians and 24-hour surgeons. I tried to see this woman more closely, my eyes unfocused from morphine, her diminuitive body a blip of browns and whites at the bottom horizon of the ceiling.

She did not wait for a nurse. She did not hesitate. There was in her a humility that did not weigh the value of one human being against another. There was no clash between what she might do for me and what she could do for herself or someone else. She left only for a minute to return with a basin of warm, soapy water and some clean towelettes. I tried to separate my weakened legs. She opened them quietly without violence or direction. I cried the cry of an infant who has her need met. So gently as to soften the edges of her broken English, she asked me about why I had come to Israel. Too confused to answer, instead I struggled to lift my hips and couldn't. She pulled the wet linens from beneath me and doubled a towel to catch the water.

I cannot begin to describe to you the deliberation with which she cleaned my body, nor the relief, comfort, and sanctification I felt as I was being cleansed. Because she was gracious and helped me to collect myself, I learned that the taking of urine and feces from another person can be a holy act. She continued silently, thoroughly, patting me dry, laying a fresh sheet, taking my hand again.

In a Minnie Mouse voice, vocal cords stretched in traction, I used the vernacular of the Jewish Orthodox, "Baruch Ha-Shem". It sounded very funny. "Baruch Ha-Shem," she smiled. Blessed is The Name. Thanks to God, for then I felt God in her. I did not feel pity but a woman's piety. I could see the nurses' disdain for bed pans and diapers without the suffering and degradation. She had taken my humiliation and helplessness in those hours and single-handedly wrangled them into well-being. It was an opportunity to "change someone" not even I could miss.

This was a major lesson of my disability, taught by a non-disabled woman in a distant land in the course of about 10-15 minutes. She taught me the beauty of laying low. Nancy Mairs, a writer with multiple sclerosis, once wrote that she wished others could see as she does from her wheelchair, "waist-high" among the non-disabled. Technically I was "gurney-high", but really my perspective was changed more earthily, crumbled to *hummus*, shifted physically and spiritually to the ground.

The injury to my cord was slight, compressing rather than cutting, so my glimpse into the conditions of death lasted during the first weeks of care while they stabilized and operated on me. My mortification about having jumped on a camel in my dehydrated, scattered state lessened as the consequences of my injury became clear. My high-flown plans for the summer and fall still absorbed me so that between toileting and napping I plotted how I could begin walking by myself and study *Torah* part-time. I don't think we can help it. We are lured back into life by what promises it seems to make to us. I dreamed of returning to the States and taking my first job as a college professor.

A month later, when my mother Ruth was helping me navigate the uneven pavement of modern West Jerusalem, I considered my own fragility, how it felt fraught with fear. I saw how my body's healing brought with it numerous, small changes that felt unknown to me when they should have felt familiar. Part of this came from having a little of that phenomenon after SCI where your head and your body all the sudden feel disconnected. How to put my head and body back together again? How would I emerge at the end of this? What change of self would be worth all I was going through? Did I get to decide? My head bobbed down the *Via Dolorosa* where Christ last walked, while my legs contemplated the distance behind like a pair of heretical commentators or Prufrock's bodiless claws scuttling across the floor of silent seas.

Another image of healing I came to nearly blew my wheels off: I thought that with each humiliation I endured, whether through cruelty, kindness, or chance, I might experience a new rebirth. I could learn what I could bear. I would relearn my own bearing. My bearing was off. Most of ours are. Most of us bumble in the world. Depending on whom you talk to, most of the world is a no-man's land. But if I stayed open to it, I might learn more through this body with disability than I could ever in a body that rarely went through noticeable change. I accepted my parents' nurturing care. I accepted the places I would not be going and the endless waiting for specialists. In each scrutinized step over cobblestone I felt the exhausted happiness of the marathon runner. Hours spent at the Israeli transportation bureau for people with disabilities felt strangely like being received by heads of state. From my lowly place I saw how each thing was important. But can humility last?

Recently I have been writing about disability after the *Intifada*, the intense conflict between Israel and Palestine that began in 1987 and resurged in 1997. The intermediacy of my injuries happened to match the "no-man's land" between warring peoples. I had been injured on disputed soil. I was stabilizing and rehabilitating in a disputed city. Our apartment literally sat on the Green Line that once divided Arab and Jewish territories. Bombers targeted our local open market and lunch place. Two days after I returned to the States I saw on the news the dead face of the same young man who had sold us ripe bananas. Near the wall where earlier my nephew had become a man, other men had attacked and occupied one of the holiest of mosques. Once my mother put her body between me and five tough boys who were chucking stones at a bearded man who scurried along the tunnel between territories. I smarted over both the skirmish and the maternal intervention. I wanted to rise up and stop the violence from happening. In sight of each other, we were all casualties.

The trauma of this time for both peoples is coincidentally ingrained in my consciousness, fused with part of my hip into my neck. The good and ill will, the humanity of the peoples of this little Holy Land, are part of me now, ground and molded into the little isthmus between my shoulders and my head. The way that some Israelis and Palestinians want to take each others' lives can send my butt muscles into spasm and my anxiety through the roof. Uncomfortably as this may sound, I feel the circumstances of the world around my ISCI in my body's make up. If they could all think just a little bit less of themselves, perhaps they would all fit in. Consider the forces that bring us to humility. Did they have to be violent to be effective? Could they be more like that hospital volunteer, whose virtue lay in reversing the effects of dirty work?

So it is particularly important for me to feel safe and sound with my body in the aftermath of my ISCI in the

Middle East. At the same time, it is important for all of us to find new contexts and new associations for our bodies, so we are not just products of someone's violence or of accident. We can look at each other's lives with spinal cord injuries, or other disabilities, or humble like-mindedness and accord each other the great liveliness we are due. As someone with ISCI, I accept that my place in the disability community now and in any disability community that we might create is tenuous. Because I don't look disabled, I go through much of my recovery without formal community or resources. I am often humilated and humbled when passed over for opportunities to grow, explore, work, or produce because I do not look hurt enough. I have been hurt enough.

It became clear to me in the years to follow, when I returned to the States and began trying to reconstruct an academic career, that very few people with SCI actually have an "SCI community" and that many of us go through the fear and transformation alone. The obstacles for those of us with ISCI who can use our arms or legs grow even heavier, since we are often left alone to move them. We must diligently construct our community and try to be inclusive of all those who need it, people with old or new injuries, people with mild or severe injury, people who bounce back and those who don't.

While our community as people with SCI doesn't need to be grand in any way, it is important that something be created out of it, some knowledge of ourselves and others that expresses our distinctiveness within the fabric of humanity, or some usefulness found in the company of others whose bodies have seen some of the same action as our own.

For folks like me whose ability to "pass" among the non-disabled masks the deeper realities of our SCI experiences, this distinction, I believe, requires us to flesh out the understanding of ISCI in both the SCI community and the disability community at large. Unlike being judged by the color of our skin, we are judged by our failure to meet norms, disabled or non-disabled. We are spared the stares and whispers, and we have neglected the importance of our difference. Because our spinal cord injuries can be experienced so differently, our ways of being are extremely diverse. Imagine looking exactly like everyone else but *being* diverse. Usually it's the opposite: we look different from most others but wish to be understood that we are the same.

Myself is more than myself. I mean this to say that my life means more than my life ever could mean to me singly. The diversity of myself—in this place, among others with disabilities—requires me never to assume that I have the line on what makes me or others tick. In this lowly state, I'm really in the best possible state of personal survival.

It's really when I acknowledge the mortal dimensions of my injury that I come to any terms with my disability. Like many of us who did not have disabilities before our SCIs, I fall into one pothole after another of default experiences. I look normal ergo I must be to some special degree non-disabled. Friends with brain injuries understand this well. I tell myself my injury is an event that once happened to me but which is now over; the actual contour of my life provides evidence that my spinal cord injury is something still happening to me every day.

I trip over this thinking left and right: rather than ending, my career leveled me to points of illumination and frustration I could never imagine. My friends mostly have academic tenure or such, while I am still balancing my colossal mental appetite with my ability to work a full day every day. I am becoming an itinerant scholar, shaped by less desire to have it all and driven still to have something. Being able to understand what that something is would probably fill another essay. Nine years after injury, I am still searching, still trying to transform humiliation into humbleness. It took me four years and three therapists simply to accept that my disability is real to me. I am a slow learner. But that's okay: my body won't give up on me. In my effort to cope with ISCI, for example, I would like to let go of difficult and excruciating memories that attend my accident. I would love sometimes to wake up every day with the same strong, happy-go-lucky body I used to have. But my psyche sends waves of anxiety through me like the errant of each detail that I would suppress. My anxiety tells me often what my body and my intellect try to forget.

There's a whole realm of disability that I am somewhat fearful to inhabit. But I am also so glad to be part of it. If I am mortified in this contested territory of experience and identity, it is only because I am truly alive and made aware of the subtler differences between life and death. The horizon between this state and the next is ever moving forward before me, and I know just enough to see the value of our humility. I keep thinking of us people with spinal cord injuries as people who have evolved, who have moved ahead. We have our heads on us. We are useful in our espousal of humility. We have the ability to speak to the most magnificent and most small of themes: losing and finding, movement and stillness. In humility we are carrying ourselves, carrying others, having ourselves carried through this mortal expanse.

8

MARC NAVARRO ON RECONNECTION

In the world of music, going to concert shows is like going to family reunions, your family increasing as you meet new performers and their listeners. I may understand these people better than I know my own family. I have always felt able to relate to these friends better, for our music helps us to get around life's complications and share our interests, as far back as I can remember. Having a spinal cord injury is every-thing but uncomplicated, however, so I have had to look for safe, enriching connections that relate two basic truths about myself: first, that I love to make and listen to music; and second, that I am now a person with a disability. When I first looked at my situation clearly, the second truth appeared to screw up the first. Here is how I accepted, through my life in music, that the difference between connecting and reconnecting with others is a difficult and intense process.

I have known Ryan Horky since he and my brother Ronnie were in seventh grade. His little brother, Craig, was one year ahead of me in sixth, but we would all hang out together at school, skateboarding and getting into fights. Since I had been playing drums since the third grade, music came before our friendships. I didn't need many lessons, just one or two. Ryan was already playing his drums. Ronnie got his electric guitar in fifth grade and we almost instantly started our band, playing off and on with other middle schoolers in mighty jam sessions at our farmhouse in the boonies of Blissfield, Michigan, houses placed neatly at every mile with cornfields in between.

Guitar World magazine had these guitar tabs, little

cheat sheets; we would try to play these songs each month, working our way through Led Zeppelin, Black Sabbath, The Who. We felt such great passion that we would cover all the musicians we could think of. For me, it was all the best drummers: John Bonham, Bill Ward, Keith Moon. They were the heaviest, playing their drums loud and fast, with cool solos I couldn't play but would try to imitate anyway, except I didn't bang around my head till later. I used to flip through my dad's records and pick out my idols. After I got bored with classic rock, heavy metal and I came into our own; we'd imitate Guns 'n' Roses, Motley Crüe, Poison, and Iron Maiden. With Craig and Ryan, I moved into grunge rock, Nirvana, Alice in Chains, Soundgarden, Pearl Jam, alternative sound, which as MTV reported, killed heavy metal.

Our friendships got tighter as we took each turn through the popular sound of the day. Whatever one of us wanted to do, we'd swing into that. We hooked up with people who shared our passion and freedom. Bob Taylor, who later became my dad's brother-in-law, and who funny enough is younger than Ronnie, became Ronnie's artistic mentor, a cool dude to hang out with. We looked up to Bob, with his reddish brown curly long hair (it was all about long, grungy hair and pierced ears back then.) Whatever Bob was into, we wanted to be into, and he brought with him the music of new bands we would not have heard otherwise, living so far out in the country.

Eye to eye with musical friends, I experienced the feeling of establishment. We were all really tight, our crowd growing to include other friends at school. Matt Dunbar and his cousin Jake Retter would play with us. We worshiped Nirvana together, figuring out their lyrics and chords, and we stuck together through our stupidity. In seventh grade Jake and I got drunk and broke into his neighbor's house, making ourselves at home and cleaning some kid's room out of CDs and video games. When Officer Pooley came to my parents' door, I was put on house arrest and given probation with a term of study at Maurice Spears Campus for juvenile delinquents. I saw one of my cousins in there. This was our lives.

After graduating high school, Ron started another

band in Saginaw called Abound Failure. Their drummer and bassist were not working out, so they asked me and our friend John Burtle to fill in at a Jamestown Hall gig in March of 1999. My buddy Mike Butler—every one called him Troll—was old enough to drive me to the gig. He was a funny, sarcastic guy who on my 16th birthday put a cheap teddy on his 200-pound body and popped out a cake. That night, we played hard and loud to a big crowd, people cheering at my crazy, spasmodic drumming, Buddy Holly prescription glasses, sweating like I stole something. We headed back to Blissfield after midnight.

Troll was driving, Justin in the front seat, John, Diego, and me comfortable, pretty much passed out, in the back of Justin's parents' Bravada. Really tired, Troll fell asleep at the wheel. We hit a guard rail and rolled five times into the embankment. Except for my neck injury, everyone else just had bumps and bruises. I was asleep for the whole thing. I remember lights as they extracted me out of the car using the Jaws of Life. Diego was pinned underneath, yelling for me to move. I couldn't. According to lore, two intoxicated women came to help us, calling 9-1-1 and Life Flight, which took me to St. Joseph's Hospital in Ann Arbor. My mother tells me that one of the paramedics from Life Flight asked after me, telling her that she could see the life in my unconscious eyes, laying her hands on me to make sure, knowing I would survive. My only memory of the first hours at the hospital was of coming to and telling them my mother's phone number.

Zoned out on narcotics, off and on I could see people in my room. I couldn't tell day from night, but Ryan, Craig, Ronnie, Troll, Diego, John, and my little brother Bubba all came out that first night to stay with my mother and father in the ICU. Every day they came, all of them sleeping over, until the hospital set limits on their visits. Some nurses knew, though, that young kids needed other young kids, so let them sneak in to see me. Justin asked me after the fact if I remembered seeing them, and I dug down deep for the memory. Like a dream reality, I couldn't tell what was real, their faces above mine, so many of them sometimes that there wasn't enough room. My parents never left.

My friends acted like they were happy to see me but were trying to hide how unsure they felt. They were trying to act normal. It felt comfortable being around family and friends in a strange place. We didn't know then how badly I was hurt, not much registering in my head between and after doctors would visit, after the swelling went down, and they did surgery. I had two different tracheotomies, and when one was removed, I could finally say it was painful. I couldn't feel my legs.

After I moved to rehabilitation at Eisenhower Center in Ann Arbor, I called Ron and everyone up to see where they stood on the band. Even if I couldn't play drums yet, I wanted to do something else, anything else, sing, write, anything musical. I felt I needed to reestablish myself through music. Everyone said let's do it we started writing pulling Josh Call in from Saginaw as our drummer. We called him Our Other Brother from Our Other Mother. Ron would pick me up and we would go down to Justin's garage to write and mess around. It was good to be in the band again, but I felt nervous about singing in public, never having been the front man

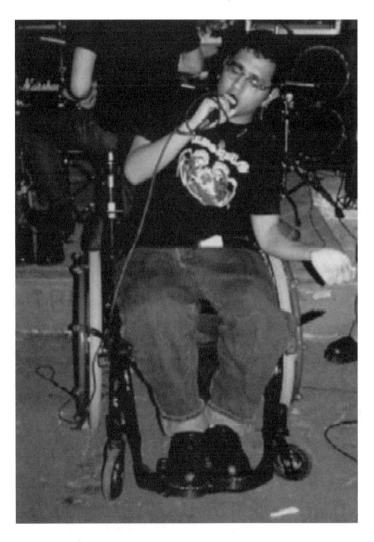

Marc Navarro performing with Tomorrow Feels Like Sunday at Who's Emma, Toronto

before. Some of it was also about being in a wheelchair. I had never seen anyone do this before in a chair so didn't know how the crowd would react.

I didn't let myself think about this a lot, telling myself I would be comfortable anywhere with my band. And the crowd—friends—liked us. I got used to it. I had to.

That first year after injury I played as I much as I could, four or five times a month, back and forth between the hell of rehab and a sweet garage in Blissfield. There was more going on in me than just the tunes I could hear. This was a place where I felt comfortable and safe in the music, both before and after my injury. Music connected both parts of my life. When you lose and find something again, it feels like opening up the kind of present that you can keep opening up and it never gets old. You can go back again and again to open it and there's always the same feeling. Like Drew Barrymore unwrapping the same video to remember her life each day in the movie *Fifty First Dates*, I connected my missed time with each time making music with my friends, never wanting to disconnect again.

Over the next few years, however, my friends started coming over less and less, maybe because they thought I had established myself and needed less support. I am not sure if I needed less support or not. Some friends became shadier than others. Perhaps they were really busy in their own lives. Perhaps they were getting bored, bored with hanging out with me, doing the same things everyday. Justin and Aaron left the band for colleges in Kalamazoo and Mount Pleasant, Troll moved to Minnesota for Bible college and got married. I would see Josh, Ryan, and Craig at shows, but we really didn't hang out after the band's deterioration. John became a tattoo artist in New York City. Diego went back to South America.

In reflection, my friends had just moved on to practical plans: career choices, schools, wives. At the time, though, I was so busy trying to keep the band together, *keeping myself together in the band*, that I lost track of who was staying and who was going. I stopped making the effort, my life falling into pieces. My girlfriend and I broke up and Ron and I tried to put together a music label without bands to play. We had too much trouble finding our own band members. Ron moved to Lansing. My parents started to divorce. Basically, it was FUBAR, if you know any Army lingo.

I haven't been in a band for almost four and a half years now, and while I think it was a good idea we all broke up, it felt like they were about to shoot Old Yeller, and I was Old Yeller. It felt awful. After the fact, I realized that we all needed this. We weren't happy any more in our relationships. I felt I had failed, that everything I had worked for had died. I went through a depression for two years, not leaving the house much, sleeping a lot, crying all the time. I thought getting it all out would make me feel better, but I ended up feeling worse.

Eight new tattoos on my body reflected the pain of that time. Inducing more pain I thought would help me forget about people. The tattoos distracted me from my depression, the feeling that I had made mistakes, breaking up the band, breaking up with my girlfriend, breaking up so many deep relationships. In 2000 I had a pair of angels tattooed on my chest, their faces looking in opposite directions, seeming to push up clouds that aren't really there. I'd modeled them off a split CD of Seasons of the Field and Pensive. They were guardians of my troubles, making sure I didn't do anything stupid, setting myself up for more failure, more disappointment.

The tattoos brought me more meaning in the months and years to follow. In one, a skeleton pulls an angel down: in this tattoo, she looks like she's giving up but also that she's fighting really hard. Like her, I struggle in my wheelchair and everything that comes with it. When I stopped and thought about things in those tough years, I began to see that what happened to me was not a bad thing. I feel more that we are fighters, this angel and I. When I am down, she looks like she is giving up. Really she's not giving up, though. She is accepting. I can look at my forearm, and she does everything that I cannot do. She can fight because I can't fight. She can fly because I can't fly. She can cry when I can't cry. She's my personal Jesus or something.

Last time I saw my old friends, we were at this big outdoor show, and I saw them from far away. I knew Ryan and Craig could see me, but they didn't come up to say hi or anything. I felt insulted and pissed off but brushed it off. I didn't need them, I told myself. They made me feel like I was a stranger or a ghost. It was like I was no longer there, expendable. Did I no longer matter to them? Did they think about me any more? Am I really unnoticeable? I've know wives to leave their husbands because they are in wheelchairs, and families to let their kids go because they are not sound of mind. This makes the rejection by my friends even worse, because there is no reason for them to forget me.

In that way, my injury is like a new life for me. The old life is over, the new life is what I have now. I don't know if they've changed since then, but I have. Now I think about how to meet new people, friends who feel that my SCI was a big deal *so* stick around. If I had won the Lotto, those friends would have stuck around. I don't need friends like those.

Recently I ran into my friend Jenny, my friend Lexzee's cousin, in line at the Blissfield Frosty Boy. I almost didn't recognize her or her little boy when she turned around in surprise and said my name. I had been thinking randomly of old friends when with a *poof*, she was right in front of me, and we fell into that sort of conversation about running into friends of friends, which in Lenawee County is not all that unusual. Where I live is fairly small. Everybody knows some-body through somebody. Everyone's connected but one's close friends come, go, and return without notice. Blink and you might miss them. Had I been turned the other way at the Frosty Boy I might never have seen this friend of mine. I have to come to terms with parting with my friends and seeing them return. While they had been there for me in the hospital and appeared devoted to my making it out of there, one by one they had disappeared. With every year, another one of my friends would cut his tie with me. It happens so quickly, too.

I think about this all the time: are they too busy living life or too stuck up or too scared to stay friends with a man with a disability? My experiences go much farther away than the common man's. I travel more distance than they may ever go. As much as I liked seeing my friends, I was also hurt by this, not by Jenny in particular; she wasn't one of the friends who would simply ignore me. I feel angrier with my band people and others who once shared with me the enjoyment of music, the most important passion of my life. It is hard not to have say over who goes and who stays, who will be my friend today with me as I am now and who will be there for me when I need them. How much of a friend is a friend? Five years ago I wrote these lyrics for our band's song "My Best Friend", the starting point of the domino effect of losing my friends, losing those I loved: "What if I died tonight?/ Would you lay by my side?/ Would you still be there?/ Would you even care?/ Look into my eyes/ Would you speak a thousand lies?" Reconnection when life crashes down is tough for everybody.

Through my disability, I became a stronger person in dealing with my everyday reality. Although I had this great tragedy, and I don't wish to deny that, I find now that life in general is full of such events. How each person deals with that everyday reality is what defines us as people. You will never find someone who hasn't experienced loss himself or known someone else who has experienced it. There are gaps all over the place, places of disconnection that require reconnection.

Yesterday, my friendly caregiver Owen and I went to Lexzee's for Easter dinner. There I thought about, sitting in that room with these newer friends, how Owen's stepdad had just committed suicide and Lexie's older sister, who would have been my age, had been killed in a car crash the Thanksgiving before my accident. Not only in my life but in theirs, so many people have these tragedies and struggle with the things I struggle with. Whether it be a family member dying or an illness of one's own, within one's own community of friends there is usually tragedy. These tragedies fade, but their places among us don't. We have to figure out how to fill that silence ourselves.

The discord of sharing our struggles in times of serious accidents or other so-called tragedies sounds better when we allow the off-key to occur, both in our lives and friendships. My accident led to my transformation. I'm not just human, but something new, like a caterpillar going through the cocoon in its ugliest and most beautiful moments. Maybe I have used music culture to express this. Strangely, I am not as dependent on popular music as I used to be, either. I was at an

August Burns Red concert recently thinking about people with injuries and disabilities, how we go through life in cruel and bitter ways, how we get ignored by the common person, how some of us get totally alienated. The music takes me to my own needs for connecting with others, and my disability returns me to the power of music in linking me to this place in my own way.

I think now that had my accident never happened I would never have met the people I have, nor would I be as strong as I am now. I also have a better understanding of true friendship, that it is something that we can't buy. True friendship is something like family. As I remember my accident, I am also able to remember my friends. My accident is stronger than many of the friendships that I lost in that my accident is something I will always have as part of who I am, whereas those friendships I really have lost. It almost makes sense now, thinking about true connection, that if those friends had been true, they would have hung around a lot longer. More than just people to make music with, they might have become people to confide in. The friends who did not stay around were part of the hand that life has dealt me. That same hand led me to another deal where I would find better friends.

I am still worried about losing the people who support me instead of depending on myself to do things. I need reconnection. So I plan to have more fun, worry less. As this is being published, I am stoked to go to the non-stop metal 2006 Robot Mosh Fest this summer in Wisconsin. Even though we have to depend on others, if we do not help ourselves out, we will sit and do nothing. Without dreams or goals to help us reach out to the world, we will amount to nothing and we will never be happy.

Why coast through life wondering "what if?" when we can connect with others on our own terms? We can look at our spinal cord injuries as obstacles dooming us to a separate existence from the rest of the earth, or we can be more than One Hit Wonders. Until others see their own connection to us, we sort of have to do our own thing, make our own music. And we must be careful about our human reconnection. For now, I find it fulfilling at least to write a song and have others like it. It is a start. There is more than one way to connect with people, and for me that is also the great thing about the making of music. It helps me at least to feel closer, to know that others will let themselves join the life inside the sound. That goes for me, too. Through words and song, I can connect with so many. That is what makes the music perfect. Those people can know exactly how I feel and still not disappear into their own fears. In my music or in theirs, we find much needed courage.

9

When I first meet you I don't know much about you.
At first glance, I sum you up. Perception is the way that
others see you or the way that you see yourself. That perception changes as I talk with you and learn your ideas. But
the way I see you may be neither how you see yourself nor
how you really are. It is human nature to judge quickly,
however inaccurately: until I get to know you, you may be
really different from the way I see you.

All of us—including those of us with spinal cord
injuries—get prejudged because of our disabilities. We're

153

such a physical society, judging people by the way we look. It happens automatically that we prejudge, often negatively so, people who use wheelchairs, crutches, or other solutions for their mobility problems. I struggle with sayings like "oh, that poor person in that chair!", for this is a sort of statement of physical prejudging that takes perception to an extreme. The people who say this often look at us as having no value, self-worth, or usefulness in the world. This is more of a social prejudging of people with disabilities as a group.

Of course, social prejudging is normal but also wrong. It is wrong for us because it's inaccurate and affects us on a bigger scale. Our culture has changed enough so that today most of us with SCI can embrace our disabilities. Still, this social prejudging keeps happening on a regular basis. Many non-disabled people are so afraid that our condition could become theirs. Perceiving us in this useless way serves an emotional and social purpose for them. They keep their minds on only one possibility for a good life, tossing phrases like "wheelchair-bound" and "crippled" around in normal conversation. They want to keep up with the Joneses with a house, a picket fence, and two kids; no one would intentionally trade that dream lifestyle for any lifestyle that jeopardizes that dream. They would not dare to imagine themselves disabled. We remind them of this. In their push for normalcy, they worry that any disruption in their plans would make them less productive or worthwhile.

Before I was injured, I used to look at people in wheelchairs and assume that there must be something wrong with their legs, and so life must really be complicated for them. I was a physical prejudger at least. I just looked at their mobility problems, without any idea of the total involvement of their injuries or who they were as people. I was a single mother working three jobs, teaching pre-school, serving customers at Sears in the evening, and selling Avon at both jobs. My children were my world and I had set my mind on the best for them.

To tell you the truth, I am not sure I was even looking at the person with SCI as a person. I did not look at people but at their injuries. I simply didn't think of them in the contexts of being people—what their work consisted of, who their families were. But in the late sixties and early seventies we got to see very few people with disabilities. The perception then was that disabled people were being institutionalized or getting stuck at home someplace.

As a healthy, strong, and particularly physical person, I never thought that this could be me. Like everyone else, I thought I don't have to think about this so didn't. There was little empathy because of my own ignorance of them and of myself. It turned out I wasn't the person I thought I was either. In 1976, traveling with my mother, brother, sister, and two young children from Michigan to California, I acquired my disability as the result of an automobile accident.

Doctors told me that my neck had been broken between the 6th and 7th vertebra, that I would be totally dependent upon others, and that I would never be able to do anything for myself. At the same time, I was given the devastating news that my son had been killed. My thoughts quickly shifted from my injuries to the safety and well-being of my daughter who was in the car as well. Even though she and my son were sitting side by side, (thank God) she received only minor injuries.

I did not really perceive myself at that time. Doctors informed me that the complete break to my spinal cord would leave me paralyzed from my shoulders down. While I was lucky to be alive, they emphasized again that I would need someone to take care of me for the rest of my life. This was their perception of me, and for what it was worth, I accepted it without question. With my son having died and my daughter injured, the total of my experience did not occur to me.

A spinal cord injury meant, more than about walking. It was a whole life change. I very quickly processed what the doctors had said. I had my father bring me a picture of my son, Eddie, Jr., as I lay on the Striker frame, so I could come to grips with his passing. My thoughts were about my remaining abilities to decipher and reason, foremost about how I could be the best parent to my remaining child, LaTronda. As I lay there in the intensive care unit not able to move, my mind began to flashback on the few people I had seen with disabilities, wondering what their lives must be like and trying to imagine my life with a disability. I began to concentrate on what I could do and on the person I still was. I realized I needed to learn as much as I could about this condition called spinal cord injury.

As reality set in, my perception of people with disabilities began to change at that moment. I needed to come to grips with the fact that life would be different for me in almost every way. "Are you sure you tightened those bolts real good?" I would ask the nurses, getting on their nerves as they turned me on my frame like a pancake. In order for us to really take control of our lives, we must actually take control. I tried to see as much as I could. I learned all about my spinal cord— how it works, how it would be affected— and found I could still have a quality of life.

I began to pray, drawing on my faith in God to help me deal with all the changes my body was going through. In order for my mind and body to work together, I also needed my soul and heart to heal. Soul and heart often reveal truths to us. We often get so concerned about walking that we forget about healing. The loss and separation were devastating, including my physical separation from the child whom I had last seen as healthy. My spirituality supported me in understanding that God does not make mistakes and that the seven years that I had with my son bore significant meaning.

God made it possible, too, for me to call my daughter each day and to look upon each day as a day to move forward. I learned that I would not need to walk in order to raise her, to lead and guide her toward becoming a healthy adult. My mom took my daughter home to live with her during the three months I was at the University of Nebraska Hospital. I realized that what I would need from rehabilitation would be things to make me stronger, to do the things I would physically need to do to make my life goals of independence and motherhood happen. This was when I developed a new perception that I could be in a chair and still be worthwhile, still do everything, just do it differently.

I insisted that the nurses give me a strap to feed myself, even though my doctors thought I would never be able to manage it. My father watched me carry three garden peas on a spoon from the plate, only one pea making it by the time it reached my mouth, crying, "Daughter, daughter, you

don't have to go through this." He didn't see the depths of
why I did this. He had seen the severity of my injuries. My
father is a Baptist minister, I should mention, who knows
about faith in God and miracles. So consumed with my
injuries, the loss of my ability to care for myself, and relying
on the doctor's poor prognosis, my father saw my wanting to
feed myself as too much effort. No parent wants to see his
child suffer and he wanted to relieve me of such suffering.

Yet the struggle and the effort, even with the losses of
my son and my bodily function, were part of the process. The
revelation came to me that even if I couldn't do it, I could re-
lay to someone what I needed done. I ate those peas because I
perceived that as something I could take control of myself.
Like in the Serenity Prayer, I accepted that I couldn't change
what happened to me, but I could change other things.
If I could get one pea to my mouth, then tomorrow maybe
I could get two. Maybe tomorrow I could also get a bite
of meat. I don't mean to sound cocky here. But I felt
confident. Often we let our setbacks completely put us back
where we were before. My pastor says my setbacks are set up

for my comeback.

My prognosis for an independent life looked better later as I began to take therapy at the Rehabilitation Institute of Michigan in downtown Detroit. After spending three months at rehab, I flew to Florida to join my parents and daughter while she completed first grade. They had the grand, protective idea that they would take care of me. They thought that I did not need to live on my own. I knew that I was going to make it. I knew I could come home, manage my own finances and care, and raise my daughter. My mother and father saw me as literally broken. They couldn't see life for me without support. It was like being a baby again, being cared for in every way. My mother would tell me that I didn't need to do things for myself. She was trying to help, her maternal instinct returning to care for her child.

But I was an adult, not a child. I had to do what was best for me and my daughter. In the disability community we call this "enablement." Most times our families don't even realize that their instincts to care for us may be hampering our recovery and growth as whole people. We are helped out of being all that we are. As with everything else we experience in adulthood, our disabilities are part of our maturation process. In actuality, I knew there would be limitations if I stayed there. I didn't love my mother and father any less. I just needed to grow. Much to my parents' dismay, we returned to our home in Michigan when her school was over. I focused on getting back there as soon as possible in order to help my daughter though this period of instability and change. I grew from a snapshot vision of myself lying on my back on the stretcher, with my daughter watching me lose it over Eddie, to a better picture of myself in her world.

Now my dad calls me his "Wonder Woman Ways" and tells me I am one of the strongest women he knows. The things I have done, the life I continue to live, the things I will do, amaze him, for he knows there's nothing I cannot do. Now I really inhabit the life my spinal cord injury has caused. My disability is normal for me. No matter what we plan to do, whether spur of the moment or a planned adventure, people around me still need to work my normal into their normal. They forget I am in a chair because they feel my worth and they know I do everything for myself and for them. They just look at my chair as a means of mobility for me. People see my chair and they also don't see it.

After LaTronda and I were going it on our own, I quickly found that attendant care wasn't necessary for me. I was able to care for myself. Taking control of my personal care had practical benefits. Trustworthy caregivers of quality are hard to find. At my place, money, jewelry, and food would often go missing. Other disabled people tell me they have been abused by caretakers but don't report it for fear of retribution. We look like sitting targets. Seeing only what they want from us can turn our lives into a nightmare. I saw that just because someone perceives my situation as one thing—vulnerable, impossible, or negative in some way—doesn't mean I have to own that.

I went about my business taking care of my child, getting her off to school in the mornings. When she got out of school, I took her to cheerleading and basketball practice. I worked with my daughter's strengths in combination with my own. I was so busy that it never dawned on me that I was doing all these things. I must be clear that my daughter was not my caregiver. I was the mom. I was her caregiver. We simply timed ourselves well, my doing my motherly duties plus cathing and transferring and other necessities in times when she would be doing other things. She would say she could help, and I would say no, you don't have to do that. LaTronda did her normal chores, but was never allowed to pass that thin line of doing my duties. In this way, we shared our responsibilities. Others look at us and say what a miracle it is that disabled parents can do the things we do, but really all we are doing is adjusting ourselves to do all the things we feel are normal. If people could just understand that we are driven by the same impulses to survive and thrive, we would all be in a much better place.

As LaTronda got older and more active in school, modeling, and pageantry, I got more involved outside the house, for her, on boards, and in volunteerism for the disability community. Again my life became so full that I was brimming over, not just existing. I was living in the moment. Other people were not. I encountered such a strangeness around the whirlwind of good things that were happening to us. At the age of ten, my daughter won her first Inkster, Michigan, preteen pageant, so we were off to New York, where she performed at the Apollo Theater. We were unstoppable, riding a joyous rollercoaster with its dips and inclines, yelling "wheeeee" with our hands up and into everything.

As my daughter had many friends and I had such a big van, I would be the mother to run the kids around and host pizza and popcorn after games. I got to be the cool mom. I didn't realize at the time that keeping her active and involved kept me active and involved. At games I would be the loudest one cheering, with others looking at the lady in the wheelchair. What is she doing there? They would literally stare. I could see a number of questions—how was this possible? How could she have an athlete child? How did she get here? Why is she interested in what's going on out there? Why does she want to be involved?—flashing across their faces. It would take them a pregnant moment to come to any realization that they were being impolite. Then they would congratulate me for my go-getter attitude when I was just being me.

For some reason they think I am inspirational. The pride I felt at being a parent wasn't of being a disabled parent until others pointed that out to me. Others saw me as some extraordinary person defying all the odds, while I saw myself as just a loving, caring mother proud of her daughter's achievements. Their own inadequacies, perhaps— not taking time to attend games or talk with their own children—fueled the perception that able-bodied society has in general about people with disabilities. They do not know what to do with the idea that we live and breathe as they do. A normal person would run their daughter around town and give her hugs, but somehow that is not expected of us. We're expected to hunch in a corner somewhere. But that is not the way it is.

Beyond perception, here is the way it is. The same things others do on their feet I do from my seat. I get up, take a bath, brush my teeth, dress myself, and slowly begin my day. Sometimes it takes a little extra effort. Sometimes it takes no effort at all. I do it without hesitation or second guessing but as a matter of fact. The way you put on your pants is different from how I do it, but how I do it is also very normal for me. I still put my pants one leg at a time.

My sister helped me to realize this. When she became a mother, she asked me to keep her newborn daughter while she returned to work. I said I couldn't, that I had this disability, and she said that I could. That she entrusted me with this little baby six weeks old, Christina Belinda, gave me the confidence that I could do it. Brand new child. I was scared at first. I didn't have good fingers, good hands. But I didn't stop to worry. When I needed a bottle of formula, or when I would run out of prepared stuff, I would open the can, sterilize the bottles, and make them ready. I might have done it differently, grasping things differently. Although I say my hands didn't work, they did work for what I needed done. I didn't watch myself or see myself as disabled. I would put a pillow and the baby in my lap and push my way from room to room. As I watched Chrissie grow from a little newborn until I first witnessed her sitting up and using her first words, I knew that nothing after SCI had been taken from me. I had been given greater gifts, the ability to be grateful for the smallest and most delicate of things, not just those things that are big, powerful, and major.

We are repeatedly given the gift of realization, that we need not do things to society's standards but how *we* can do it. We do not need to feel stopped because we are not standard. That doesn't mean that we are below standard. And it doesn't mean we are better than anyone else in society. Standards are entirely a matter of perception. I learned that one's perception doesn't have to be one's reality. Here I was raising, not only my own daughter but also another tiny new life. Here was the realization, somewhat like an awakening, that God's power was my reality. For me the mantra from my Christianity became "I can do all things through Christ, Jesus, who strengthens me." This was and still is my reality.

Not everyone finds the right mantra, but it means the difference between productivity and lack thereof. It means the difference between giving and receiving, the insides and the outsides of our existence together here on Earth. It means the differences between choices and chances. You can look at the abusive caregiver or staring high school parent in the eye and make choices about who you are and how you act, in God's eyes. These eyes are certainly keener than any of ours. Our lives are also not left to chance, not left to whether or not someone treats us with respect that day or understands our lives with disabilities.

We are strengthened to live independently because of the gifts we are given, far beyond the movement of our legs. I find I can play basketball table tennis, do the shot-putt, any sport I put my mind to. I have participated in them at the local, national, and international levels for most of my life, twenty-three years from my wheelchair. I stopped being a spectator on the sidelines and actively chose to play the game. Not to toot my own horn, but I have been inducted into Athletes with Disabilities Hall of Fame, an honor I feel because it recognizes people who involve themselves in the community, who think beyond just what they look like out there on the field. I now see myself very carefully. What was once true for my high schooler is true for all of us, that getting involved in sports, with its camaraderie and healthy competition, leads to getting active in the social and political arenas of our community. Instead of being someone's poster child, we become greater than ourselves.

When I applied for a position as a peer counselor at the Great Lakes Center for Independent Living (CIL), my friend Joyce Chen, another woman with a disability, also expressed amazement that I lived by myself, but I explained that no man is an island. There's no such thing as living completely by oneself or complete independent living. That is another common misconception that people with disabilities try to bear. Living independently varies from person to person. No one can live by himself. Everyone has needs to be met. Who criticizes the rich mansion dwellers for their nannies and butlers? We tend to run from one extreme to the other in our judgment of each other's independencies.

My advocacy work in the disability community began to take shape around the time of this conversation with Joyce. With the passage of the ADA, I perceived that laws needed to be enforced as well as passed. We were not receiving our full civil rights, human rights, or disability rights in housing, employment, and health care. I advocate for Money Follows the Person and MiCASSA (Medicaid Attendant Service and Supports Act) because these programs allow people with disabilities to live in their own homes in the community and receive the services and support that they need. It is only thought we are served best in nursing homes when in reality this is rarely the case. We are just perceived as too difficult or expensive to live in regular places. Health and Human Services statistics have shown that it is more economical for people to live in the community as opposed to living in nursing homes. It is about having choices that most people take for granted and that we lose first.

When it comes to the perception of people with disabilities, the only one that matters is your own. Even though we are categorized together, tetraplegics with other tetraplegics, paraplegics with other paraplegics, or amputees with other amputees, all people with disabilities are different because people are different. Each has to be viewed for his own individualism. Point in fact: two women may have a C6 injury, with doctors telling them that with this level of SCI they will be not able to do this, this, and this. For one woman, maybe a forty-year-old with more of life's seasoning, will be more tenacious in her pursuit for independence. For her the injury is a whole new adventure in which she will learn new and exciting things. She realizes that it is up to her to experience her own limits so that she sets them. At the same time she knows that there is no limit not worth attempting.

Her non-defeatist attitude will exceed everyone's perceptions and expectations, while the other woman, maybe a twenty-something who hasn't experienced life or is used to having others giving her things, will see herself as having even less potential than her doctors foresee. She will feel she needs the attendant to feed, bathe, and dress her. She will require twenty-four hour care. She gets complete dependence into her head, so she doesn't even try. She is defeated not determined. Sure enough, there will be barriers and stumbling blocks, but the forty-year-old turns those barriers into bridges, stumbling blocks into stepping stones (level ones, the kind that wheelchairs can go over), and tragedy into triumph.

How you project or how you see or feel yourself is

how others will tend to see you. If you are confident, with high self-esteem, positive thinking, and determination, others will likely see you that way. If you are uncertain, with low self-esteem, negativity, doubt, or feelings of unworthiness, then others will tend to see you that way. As Proverbs states, "As a man thinketh in his heart so is he." And as the pastor William Arthur Ward says, "If you believe it, you can achieve it." If you think you can, then you most likely will, and you think you can't, then you are defeated before you ever start. You won't make that attempt to try harder. Most people perceive people with disabilities as not having any quality of life or no life at all.

To some, it just appears easier for us to put an end to our lives. I am a member of the group called Not Dead Yet. When Jack Kevorkian was assisting people with suicide, most of his victims were people with disabilities, people who were somehow convinced that they were better off dead. I stand with Not Dead Yet in order to point out the weak values that go into prejudging people with disabilities in this sad group. In court, if an able-bodied person is having a bad day, having financial problems, even dealing with his depression, we do not suggest he commit suicide. We will do everything within our power and then some to save his life, even though he doesn't want to be saved.

It may seem easier for many people if we don't exist. The perception is that people with disabilities are these poor, pitiful, sad people who are mentally and physically trapped inside broken bodies and are desperate to be free. We are seen as bound, constrained, needing to be freed from all these unknown things that are holding us back.

For a few of us, we become convinced, usually by people without our disabilities, that life is not worth living, because we use a respirator or a wheelchair, because we use an attendant, or because we may be in constant pain. Others have decided that our life is too hard, and we have come to believe them. Yet their perception is too simplistic. They take on a "responsibility" to tell us that our lives are hard and that our disabilities are unjust, even through the truth is that it is our responsibility to lead our lives. If more of us would we take on this responsibility, the court of justice would allow people with disabilities to take more control of our own lives and be less likely to force a faulty perception on us. Rather they would support us in decisions that are sometimes difficult.

It cannot be emphasized enough that we need to be allowed to make these choices ourselves. It is usually *someone else's* perception that they have the right to tell us that we are too crippled to achieve a worthy life. The difference between this and being empathetic and compassionate is that in the latter, I am being supportive of you in the decisions you are making. I am not imposing my views on you, my thoughts, my ideas, even though I may not agree with you. You have the right and the responsibility to make your own choices, and I have a right and an obligation to support you.

It is even worse if you have a hidden disability. Even though I am member of the disability community, and I am a believer in disability culture, I too was guilty of the same preconceptions. You would think that I would have awakened to this when I was disabled myself, but the rude truth of this is that I learned this when I finally allowed myself to interact with one of my colleagues at the Center who had a profound cerebral palsy, so severe that she would communicate with a keyboard. Formerly I hadn't been willing to take the time and energy to talk with her, for her spasms made it difficult for me to maintain the conversation with speed or clarity.

When I faced this reluctance of mine and finally sat with my friend (amazing now that I could treat a friend like that) to conduct a real talk with her, I saw that she was one of the most brilliant people I had ever met. I had shocked myself not only with finally seeing her intelligence but also seeing my own severe, rude misjudgment of her, my previous unwillingness to engage her. Not that every person with a disability that I would meet would be brilliant, but I had not given myself the chance to know who she was and what she was about. Those of us with disabilities need to embrace all disabilities, not just the ones occurring from our injuries, but the whole of disability culture, people with cerebral palsy or spina bifida, multiple sclerosis, muscular dystrophy, mental illness, Tourettes syndrome, heart condition, or invisible conditions like hearing or visual impairment. See and embrace ourselves, all.

I've been fortunate to own my own business in disability transportation as well as work for the CIL and as faculty coordinator for Independence University. Afforded tremendous opportunities, I have traveled to faraway places and met famous intellectuals like Cornel West. There has never been a time when my van has broken down and some angel hasn't come to my rescue. I do not take my good fortune as a person with SCI for granted. We have a responsibility and obligation to inform and educate our brothers and sisters in the disability community. We need to come to the Center and see others like themselves working, socializing, building families, and struggling, just living our lives. They will realize that they, too, will do the same.

Before I had my disability, I would think people in wheelchairs must have something wrong with their legs. After my SCI, I saw that disability is a whole experience, including mind, body, and spirit. It's also important to perceive that people with SCI are just people, not superheroes and not poor invalids. Just people. Just like regular people, we can be a bitch or a blessing. But when people without disabilities continue to look at us with their own sort of visual disability, they are disabled from seeing us or themselves as wholes. They will continue to formulate their notions of whom we are, and what we are about, and what our values are.

When many non-disabled people look at us, they fear that our imperfections, our deformities, our deficiencies will become part of them. Sometimes we do this to ourselves. They fail to understand or comprehend that those very things may make us strong, make us wise, make us determined, make us the victor instead of the victim—these are the things that define us, that make us who we are.

Maybe they are afraid to face their own fear that we already are in them, and that they are in us, so that we must share and rebuild our society for us both. Everyone has value. Everyone has purpose. Our purpose is not rightly measured by the way he or she looks or by the way you want to see them. I have taken this to heart when I am called upon to talk to people who are newly injured, because when I see them I remind them they are just as worthy as I am. That is the secret of my success. Value, potential, and purpose are things we all have. This perception has allowed me to live a very happy, healthy, and fulfilled life. And as Jill Scott sings, I live this life like it's golden.

10

JULIE HARRISON ON PATIENCE

Note: *The following essay has been edited based on the drafts Julie Harrison left behind on the topic she had chosen to discuss for this volume. She used several methods in writing her work: she talked and wrote freely in creative fusion with her friends. She could also be immensely private and autonomous in her writing. She told us that writing about her life following spinal cord injury was important and harder than she had anticipated, especially considering that she was a researcher herself of women with spinal cord injury and other disabilities. On her journey of writing about patience she carried with her reflections of other writers, visionaries, and activists who influenced her thoughts on what patience means. Since one of us took notes with Julie, and since Julie took notes with us during our authorship sessions, we had in our hands a somewhat alluring dialogue on the subject. We felt a great depth of perspective about Julie in relation to her concerns about patience, both as a young woman and as a person with spinal cord injury. Because we respect her expression in these notes, and because she was excited to write this piece, we were tempted to "reconstruct" or "complete" or "finesse" our dialogue to augment her "voice" on the subject. After all, we knew her and one of us had been a witness and friend to her writing. To be true to the authorial process, however, none of this dialogue is reconstructed here. We feel that it is more important for Julie's readers to have just her words and her inspirations without either posthumous sentiment or mediation. It remains important for people with disabilities to have our say without distortion or "unauthorized" (re)tellings. It was a final communication on patience, since we will have to wait interminably for Julie Harrison's full exposition on the theme. But we would rather wait than interrupt her, spiritually or ethically. We agree with her that "nothing is lacking." As in all good praxis, we provide what we can rely on, leave readers to validate it as they see fit, and hope that Julie Harrison's task on patience may be picked up by another person whose knowledge extends her own.*

M.E. and T.P.

Writing is an art of telling and not telling. I dedicate this essay to "Josephine Schmo", that plain, beautiful person with spinal cord injury who sees her life in light and darks, subtle, like chiaroscuro.

J.H.

A good friend of mine likes to complain jokingly to me that I remind him of that little girl Veronica Salt in *Charlie and the Chocolate Factory.* She is one of the lucky children who win a tour of the factory. When the little "Oompa Loompas" begin waddling through, she announces to her daddy that she must take home "one of those". When he calmly explains to her that these men aren't for sale, she screams back at him, "But, Daddy, I want an Oompa Loompa and I want it NOW!" She goes on to pout. She simmers in discontent while the rest of the world goes on.

How do we learn patience as children? I am an only child. Besides getting lots of attention from my loving parents, I also got Baskin Robbins, Happy Meals, and many of the toys I wrote out on my Christmas list to Santa. With these attentive, loving parents, I grew up knowing that timing was everything. I would state my needs, wants, desires, and fulfillment of them usually would come relatively soon after. I got used to getting what I wanted.

Do not get me wrong. I may have been spoiled but I was not rotten. My parents were the authoritarian sort and I developed a healthy, mutual respect with them. They disciplined me for sassing back to my mom in the kitchen, for example, by disallowing me to attend a girlfriend's sleepover. If I kept misbehaving, I would slowly lose my privileges for fun things but never without a warning. I was given room for self-correction and the adjustment of my attitude. When I disciplined myself, I grew patient.

There is immediacy in us and there is patience. What is the secret to patience? That we can have them both, even though people think we are either patient *or* immediate. We even think of Patience as *versus* Immediacy.

You have the opportunity to recover a fresh and dynamic aliveness at the heart of your life. And aliveness means the presence of passion and spontaneity, two qualities noticeably absent in the world of judgment. It also means the experience of yourself as a life source. Life flows from and through you, taking on both familiar and unfamiliar forms. The soul's aliveness is the sense of something conscious and unpredictable, awake and mysterious.

Byron Brown, Soul without Shame

Patience is ALIVE.

Patience can really be felt when we cath. When I first had my SCI I had what I call the "rush" period. I wanted to rush through everything, get everything done. I wouldn't spend a moment more than I had to on my body and what now I needed to do for it. Now I could mediate on cathing, while cathing. I would write a "meditation on love and catheters." Just staying present and letting every moment be filled with the joy of being alive. Not rushing.

Patience is a virtue. *La verité.*

If patience is a seed in me, it has been one of the most nurtured and nourished qualities in my life post-spinal cord injury. Having patience now is a form of self-discipline I have found through writing, meditation, and diet. There is always something to be grateful for, wrote Haju. Nothing is lacking. There is nothing to worry about.

Sometime I will need to write a prayer for being present in the moment. Moments gain momentum. Watch them and they are in motion. I am the spirit of my old-woman self. I reminisce about days in my youth spent dancing on cobblestone streets in Malaga, Spain.

Innovative, spontaneous, tough, and playful, she guides us. . . helping us to cultivate awareness, relax into the body, observe the sensations, quiet the mind.

Boann, on sage teacher Ruth Denison

Julie Harrison

I go down into the musty cellar-like room
To retrieve an armful of small clay pots
Some dry and cracked like weathered skin
Spider webs catch my hair
Under the bare light bulb
Dangling from the ceiling
But this is nature I think to myself
And stay calm
Upstairs I soak the pots in water
To loosen the soil
And scrub them with a scouring pad
And rinse them in bleach-water
I stack the bathed pots to dry in the sun
Then I go downstairs for more
I do this for three hours.
                    Julie Harrison, "Washing Clay Pots"

ACKNOWLEDGMENTS

We are grateful to more people and organizations that we can record here. First and foremost we acknowledge our readers who have spinal cord injuries and who share our lived experiences. We feel that many of our authors have become our friends (not always the result of collaboration and publishing!) We thank them and their families for diligent participation and meaningful authority on so much of life, including spinal cord injury. We are grateful to the University of Michigan Model SCI Care System for their support of this project, in particular the progressive mentorship of Denise Tate, the kind editorial support of Mary Burton and Jane Walters, the able supervision of Claire Kalpakjian, and the secretarial can-do of Kay Morefield. A generous grant from the U.S. Department of Education/OSERS National Institute for Disability Research and Rehabilitation made our research into disability narratives and spinal cord injury possible. Our work found a home in the Advanced Training in Rehabilitation Research Program, seasoned well by our UM colleagues Kathie Albright, Cathy Donnell, Anthony Lequerica, and Heidi Haapala and allies in narrative research at the Rehabilitation Institute of Michigan, Colette Duggan and Tara Jeji. Influencing our search for balance between scientific and cultural understandings of disability, Sunny Roller, Els Nieuwenhuijsen, Barbara Schoen, and Julie Harrison regularly offered their expertise. Our research assistant Julianne Bonta was indispensable to *Deep*'s production. The Ann Arbor Center for Independent Living continues to inspire us.

Travar Pettway would like to thank his mother Johnnie Mae Pettway for holding him up when it felt hard to stand. Marcy Epstein thanks her parents, Ruth and Seymour Epstein, and her siblings, Nadine, Donald, and Michael, for their tireless love.